'I have been talking to patients about Appetite Retraining. This simple message has had amazing results already! Several patients have also noticed the benefits of the positive acceptance of how they feel, tuning into and trusting their deeper sensory mechanisms extending beyond their dietary habits. It took a fraction of the time to discuss and did not feel like a finger-wagging exercise on my part.'

Dr Ashish Bhatia
NHS GP

'In a world of soaring obesity, and no consensus on the best diet to follow, Helen's approach is invaluable to help our patients adopt sensible eating habits. I have used it on a personal and professional level.'

Dr Lynn Thompson
NHS GP

'Dr Helen McCarthy's individualised approach helping people struggling with weight loss and eating issues is truly unique and highly effective. I have recommended her to many of my general practice patients and only ever received excellent feedback. I have been wishing for her to write a book for a very long time in order to help bring her approach to a much wider audience.'

Dr Wolfgang Walter,
NHS GP, acupuncturist and Int
Medicine Specialist

D1113593

'I am very grateful for the way in which Dr Helen has completely transformed my approach to food. I'm no longer frightened by biscuits and chocolate. I can have biscuits in the house and leave them which I couldn't do before. I don't feel fat any more and I feel proud of myself; it's liberating.'

Carys, aged 62, politician

'I'm now more relaxed around food and no longer feel it controls my life. My confidence has increased a lot and I'm a lot happier than I was before. I didn't feel like I was on a diet because Appetite Retraining™ isn't based on calories or measuring things. Conventional diets only work short-term; this approach works more slowly but for your whole life.'

Zoe, aged 26, medical receptionist

'I was drinking far too much. My doctor told me that the drinking was causing steady weight gain, and that the weight was contributing to pain in my knees. It got to the point where my wife threatened to leave me unless I cut down dramatically. Appetite Retraining™ has changed my mindset and since losing over a stone, I don't feel any pain in my knees. I feel better in myself and can wear shirts I haven't worn for years.'

Gareth, aged 41, factory manager

'Now I can stop eating when I'm full. If I have an evening where it's a bit of a struggle, I have a rational conversation in my head. I'm thinking more about what I'm eating and find

I can manage feeling hungry in the afternoon. My fitness has improved and I get much less heartburn. What works for me is eating three times a day, which I didn't do before. I enjoy my meals and now feel the right weight.'

Richard, aged 42, business manager

'Losing weight is never easy, but with Appetite Retraining™ my husband and I can still go out for really nice meals. Retraining your appetite means not eating unless you're hungry so you do eat less, but you don't get extremely hungry… in effect, calorie counting and Appetite Retraining™ come to the same thing of eating less, but calorie counting is harder and no fun.'

Clare, aged 54, scientist

'I'm amazed how much less I'm eating. It makes such a difference knowing that you can indulge in alcohol, pastries and chocolate from time to time without feeling guilty. We have learned to eat less food which means our food bill has been reduced considerably. I can honestly say that losing this weight has been a straightforward exercise with no suffering.'

Rob, aged 57, solicitor

'I had been trying for years to lose the extra pounds that kept creeping on and never managed to shift them. With Appetite Retraining™ something just clicked.'

Anna, aged 52, writer

For Gerard, Betsy and Edward

How to
Retrain
Your
Appetite

First published in the United Kingdom in 2019 by
Pavilion
43 Great Ormond Street
London WC1N 3HZ

ISBN 978-1-91162-447-9

A CIP catalogue record for this book is available from the British Library

10 9 8 7 6 5 4 3 2

Printed and bound by IMAK Ofset, Turkey

www.pavilionbooks.com

Neither the author nor the publisher can accept responsibility for any
injury or illness that may arise as a result of following the advice contained
in this work. Any application of the information contained in the book is
at the reader's sole discretion.

This is a self-help book and does not constitute specific psychological or
medical advice. If you are unsure about anything to do with your own
weight-loss plan, please consult your doctor or otherwise seek professional,
medical advice.

If you are suffering from an eating disorder, please use this programme in
collaboration with your therapist or doctor. If you are diabetic, please use
this programme in collaboration with your diabetic nurse or doctor.

How to
Retrain
Your
Appetite

Lose weight permanently eating
everything you love

Dr Helen McCarthy
THE APPETITE DOCTOR®

COLLINS & BROWN

CONTENTS

—

INTRODUCTION

———

I'm Dr Helen McCarthy, The Appetite Doctor®. Welcome to my groundbreaking Appetite Retraining Programme, which will enable you to throw away your diet books and instead achieve permanent weight loss by changing your eating habits.

Losing weight is hard however you do it. And, for many, the hardest part is keeping the weight off after reaching their goal. I've heard many people talk about regaining weight after dieting as though it's a personal failing. It's not. Regaining weight is inevitable if the way you eat on a diet is unsustainable. Appetite Retraining is a whole new approach to weight loss that focuses, from the word go, on making it easy to stick to your goal by replacing old unhelpful eating habits with new ones that allow your body to lose weight naturally.

When you lose weight by adapting your eating habits, the change is permanent and it is easy to keep the weight off. And although it is hard work, undoing unhealthy eating habits is achievable. This book shows you how. We start with where you are now, identify the ways you eat out of tune with your body, anticipate what mental blocks might get in your way and make changes one step at a time.

About me

When it comes to the psychology of eating and weight loss, I know what I'm talking about both professionally and personally. After gaining a B.Sc. degree in Experimental Psychology at Durham University, I spent five years at Oxford University doing a doctorate in the psychology of eating disorders. After that I trained as a Clinical Psychologist in the NHS. Working in an exciting and inspiring NHS Clinical Psychology department, I learned about working with people who have mental health problems, from anxiety to depression to eating disorders, and how to try to help them. Eventually I moved to private practice and am now an Associate Fellow of the British Psychological Society and a Visiting Research Fellow at the University of Bristol. Throughout the years since I qualified in 1989, what I've loved most of all is putting what's known from the academic study of psychology into practice to help people overcome their problems.

I've lived and breathed the psychology of eating and weight loss since beginning work on it in 2011. Thousands of hours' work in mainstream Clinical Psychology and more recently in the psychology of eating and appetite, Appetite Retraining is a distillation of everything I've discovered – the result of thousands of hours of reading and helping people to use psychological techniques to return to eating in tune with their body.

www.theappetitedoctor.co.uk

Where it all began

One hot afternoon in the summer of 2011, my client Megan's final session of treatment was coming to an end. At the age of 40, Megan had developed bulimia nervosa, which had been triggered by trying to lose weight using a very low calorie meal replacement programme. I had treated her bulimia successfully using cognitive behavioural therapy.

Megan was relieved and delighted to have made such a positive recovery and thanked me as she left the room. On her way out she turned and said, 'I just wish I could lose another stone in weight.' I was stunned. I had been able, as a Clinical Psychologist, to help Megan overcome a serious eating disorder, but I had no idea how to help her simply lose a stone. Not least because I was a stone and a half heavier than I wanted to be and my own (albeit half-hearted) attempts to lose weight hadn't got very far.

Once Megan's throwaway remark woke me up to the fact that all of my Clinical Psychology training and experience wasn't up to the job of helping people lose even a moderate amount of weight, I was like a dog with a bone. I had no idea whether I could succeed, but I decided to use myself as a guinea pig and set myself the goal of losing a stone over the next four months.

The first obstacle was a holiday to the South of France the following week. My weight-loss foods were going to have to include French cheese, baguettes, pains aux raisins and chilled rosé wine, because as well as the sun and the sea, that's what

I was going on holiday for. I figured that if I adjusted *how much* of these I ate, I'd be able to start losing weight on my version of the Mediterranean diet.

I rapidly discovered that when I ate less at a meal, I was hungry again by the next. Not rocket science, but I hadn't taken much notice of whether I was hungry for as long as I could remember. Feeling hungry felt scary at first, so I had to learn how not to feel anxious about it. I soon realized that the key was to work with, not against, my bodily systems which had evolved to govern appetite and eating.

Experimenting with a mixture of conventional and cutting-edge psychological techniques, in six months I lost a stone and a half. Although it took effort and focus to lose the weight, maintaining it was easy and I have kept it off ever since.

How this book will help you

By following my Appetite Retraining Programme you will change your eating habits and lose weight. What you weigh is the result of those habits. It's what and how you eat day-in, day-out that determines your weight and whether it is increasing, decreasing or stable.

Remember that it's not eating one overly large meal that makes you gain weight, any more than skipping one meal makes you lose weight. It's your *regular* eating habits that make you the weight you are now. In this programme I will help you to identify which specific unhelpful eating habits are keeping you stuck at your current weight and work out a plan for how to change them, one at a time.

Each one of the changes you make will involve learning, step-by-step, how to use your body's natural hunger and fullness signals to guide your eating, just as you did as an infant.

You'll rediscover how to feel in control around food and eating. You'll learn how to use mild, gentle hunger every day to lose weight. By learning to allow yourself to get slightly hungry, you'll rediscover just how fantastic your favourite foods really can taste. You're likely to find that when your taste buds are at their most sensitive (that is, when you are hungry), you fancy simpler foods. Real foods.

You won't need as many high-salt, high-fat and high-sugar snacks if you only eat when you're hungry. Those snacks have been designed by food technologists to be super-tasty and are the only ones you're likely to get much taste from when you aren't hungry. But if what you really fancy when you are ready to eat is a ready-meal or fast food, or a bag of crisps or bar of chocolate, then you'll have that, and really enjoy it. Unlike diets, this programme isn't about denying yourself the foods you love.

You may have come to think of hunger as scary. I did. Feeling scared of feeling hungry meant that if I didn't know when my next meal would be, I'd eat more to avoid being hungry later. This led to eating all sorts of unnecessary calories. I'd take a Kit Kat on a train journey in case I got hungry. And if I didn't get hungry, the Kit Kat would call to me until I ate it, which I invariably did.

My programme includes anxiety management techniques that can help you overcome your fear of feeling hungry, so that you discover that you can wait to eat, just like that slim-and-in-control person you know (and rather envy). Once you've overcome that fear, you'll be free to allow yourself to wait to eat until you're hungry. And remember, that's when food tastes most fabulous.

With Appetite Retraining you'll:

» Start where you are now
» Listen to your body
» Take manageable steps
» Address mental blocks as you go

Using this book

While it may be tempting to skip to the solutions, this programme isn't about quick fixes. You will benefit from reading the earlier chapters, which give you an understanding of how your appetite system works and how your bad habits have developed. Here's a guide to what you'll find in each chapter.

Chapter 1: Understand how you developed bad eating habits in the first place and why your weight-loss attempts have failed so far.

Chapter 2: Discover how your appetite system works and how to tune into it.

Chapter 3: Learn about the psychology of eating and appetite and work out what habits you need to change.

Chapter 4: Find out how to use the Appetite Pendulum™ to learn how to stop eating when you're just full.

Chapter 5: Discover how to establish a new eating routine that enables you to eat in tune with your body and your lifestyle.

Chapter 6: Anticipate and deal with any mental blocks – saboteurs – that can get in the way of permanent weight loss, and strengthen your motivation to change.

Chapter 7: Learn to identify non-hungry eating so that you're only eating when you're definitely hungry.

Chapter 8: Understand and tackle emotional eating.

Chapter 9: Learn how to gauge what to eat, at home and
when eating out.

Chapter 10: Learn how to maintain your new weight and
stay on track.

'Most diet books tell you how to avoid
being hungry. Appetite Retraining shows
you how mild hunger is absolutely your
greatest ally when it comes to enjoying
food and losing weight.'

My manifesto for permanent weight loss

» Losing weight takes focus and effort, and I believe that you should only go through that hard work once.

» To achieve permanent weight change you need to change your eating habits permanently.

» Weight loss can, and should, be gently achieved. Brutal eating or exercise regimes should be outlawed.

» Changing eating habits means taking one step at a time, starting from how you eat now. Unlike most diets, it does NOT mean overhauling how you eat overnight.

» Meal and snack times have to fit around your lifestyle.

» Everything you eat should be real food, nothing that's been doctored to be artificially lower in calories.

» What you eat should be the foods you already love, perhaps with some new discoveries.

» When you know what foods are good for you, it's not nutritional advice you need; it's psychological advice about how to eat what and how much your body actually needs.

» Mild gentle hunger every day is your greatest ally when it comes to losing weight.

» Weight loss can, and should, be joyful and increase your self-confidence and self-esteem.

Good luck and I hope you enjoy this whole new way of eating and the results that it brings!

CHAPTER 1

—

A New Approach to Weight Loss

We all ate in tune with our bodies when we were very young. As a baby, food was just food. Babies cry when they feel hungry and when they are fed, they stop crying. They feed and then they stop. If you give babies food when they're not hungry, they turn away, not interested. Trying to cajole them into finishing what you intended to give them is a messy business. They aren't persuadable and they clamp their mouth shut, not caring where the food ends up – on the floor, over the wall, up their nose. They are using the self-regulating system of eating when hungry and stopping when full. Of course, if a pot of their favourite dessert appears it's a whole new ball game thanks to taste-specific satiety (more on this later).

For some people, eating stays pretty much like that as they grow into children and then adults. It doesn't mean they don't enjoy food. It just means that they use food to satisfy their appetite and then they stop and get on with their day. 'If only I was like that!' you may think. Well, you can be. By re-learning to eat in tune with your natural hunger and fullness signals, you can learn to stop eating when you've had just enough. And you can organize your eating routine to fit around your lifestyle, in such a way that you allow yourself to get hungry by each meal.

That's what this book is all about. It's a how-to guide full of information about how you can return to eating as you did as an infant. Without the mess.

What went wrong!

You gained weight when you stopped using your natural hunger and fullness signals to guide your eating. This can happen for many different reasons. How many of the following bad habits do you recognize in yourself?

» Finishing what's on your plate regardless of whether you're full.

» Eating what someone else has left on their plate.

» Abandoning regular mealtimes.

» Dealing with stress, distress or boredom by eating.

» Eating as a way of rebelling against someone who tells you not to.

» Using chocolate as a legal high.

» Secretly eating foods you feel you shouldn't be eating.

» Grazing on foods you just happen to see at home or work.

» Eating to keep someone else happy because they're eating or because they cooked something for you.

» Eating biscuits with coffee, or salted nuts with wine, out of habit.

» Over-reacting to the freedom of leaving home by overeating just because you can.

» 'Eating for two' during pregnancy.

» Failing to change the amount you eat when your lifestyle changes, such as leaving an active job for a sedentary one.

» Failing to adjust the amount you eat as you get older.

» Using food as a friend.

When any of these habits becomes established, we gain weight. How much we gain depends partly on how much extra food we're consuming and partly on how our bodies deal with the extra food. Because we're all different, some of us gain weight more easily and the 'bad' habits have bigger consequences for our size. Your Unhelpful Eating Habits (UEHs) are directly related to those extra pounds you want to lose.

One of my clients' first step in losing weight was to stop raiding his children's sweetie cupboard every evening during the advert break of *Coronation Street*. He was surprised to find that by just making this one change he lost half a stone, most of which came off his middle. If he'd gone back to his nightly chocolate fix, the weight would have gone back on.

'The food that your body couldn't use because it didn't need gets converted into fat, leading to excess weight. Appetite Retraining helps you declutter your eating habits so you get rid of unnecessary eating and excess pounds.'

What is Appetite Retraining?

Over the years you've accumulated Unhelpful Eating Habits
(UEHs) that involve eating more than your body needs.
With Appetite Retraining you identify what your specific
UEHs are and then you change them one at a time. Step
by step you learn to eat in tune with your body. When you
change one UEH, such as reducing the size of your evening
meal, you see something like this:

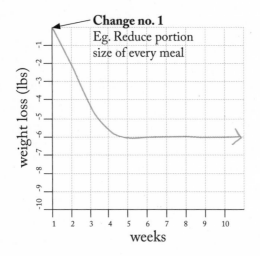

Your weight falls as you establish the new habit. And then it
plateaus. Your body has let go of the additional weight it was
carrying because of this particular eating habit. The size of the
drop in weight is something you discover, not something you
can predict. If you then reduce the size of your meals further,
you'd see an additional drop. The time to get to a plateau
depends on how big a habit change you've made and on your
metabolism. If you just make this one change and stick to it,
your weight is likely to stay around this level. To lose more,

you choose another UEH and work on making that particular change. Here's what that might look like, using the example of changing a habit of grazing on biscuits at work.

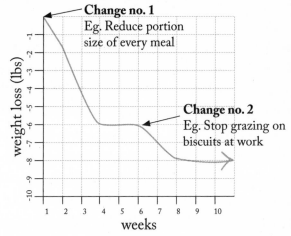

You decide how many habit changes to make, and you'll find the right balance between making changes to how you eat and what weight loss you're comfortable with.

The role of exercise

Exercise does, of course, have a role to play in weight loss, but I probably wrote a book about changing eating habits rather than increasing your activity levels because I'm not one of life's great exercisers. However, I found that when I lost weight, I wanted to move more. I joined a gym and started walking more. Not because I thought I should, but because I wanted to. When you feel better in your body you may find the same thing – that your body wants to do more.

The role of dieting in gaining weight

You may have discovered for yourself that dieting is not all it's cracked up to be. Changing what you eat and how much you eat overnight is less a recipe for success and more a sure-fire route to stress and strain around food and eating. You were already stressed about it, and adding to this is not going to work. You probably wouldn't be reading this book if it had.

The 'what the hell' effect coined by psychologists Herman and Polivy in the 1980s refers to the way dieters tend to eat unrestrainedly once they have broken a diet rule they were following. Studies have shown that it's the idea of having broken a diet rather than the amount of 'forbidden' food they consume that makes the difference. If you recognize yourself as a 'what the hell' sort of person, dieting rules are likely to lead to you eating more rather than less, and Appetite Retraining may be just what you're looking for because the focus is on habit change, not following a set of diet rules.

One of the big selling points of diet books is the 'delicious' recipes. Well, not one recipe in any diet book I've ever seen (and I've read scores of them) is as delicious as my homemade lasagne or coq au vin using the recipes in my favourite cookery book Hopkinson and Bareham's *The Prawn Cocktail Years*. So in this book, where we're talking about eating in tune with your body for the rest of your life, you won't find any recipes. You'll eat what you already love, perhaps with some new discoveries.

When you choose what to eat, and you choose the best possible version of that food, you'll get the most enjoyment from it – whether that's following Mary Berry using butter or Delia Smith using meat with fat on. Mary and Delia have been saying this for decades, despite the low-fat hysteria that has gripped the West. Call me ahead of the curve on full-fat, but that would be flattering me. I've never chosen full-fat because I thought it was healthier than low fat; I've chosen it because reduced-fat foods don't taste that good to me.

The new enemy as you may be aware isn't fat, but carbohydrates, particularly sugar. I don't know where the low-carb movement will end up as it is still the subject of fierce debate. There are impressive findings of people who dramatically reduced their carbohydrate intake going into remission from Type 2 diabetes as well as losing weight. But the movement has its more extreme elements and I am deeply sceptical about any approach that advises you not to eat too much fresh fruit. It gives me a strong feeling of déjà vu from the 1980s' advice that avocados and nuts were to be avoided because they are high in fat. Two of our current superfoods were, merely 30 years ago, to be avoided!

If you're following a diet that requires you to eat less-than-fabulous foods, you're always going to be missing out on the most pleasurable food. Whereas if you eat all of your favourite foods, and learn to eat just as much of them as your body needs at each meal, you'll never be missing out. Except on the less-tasty foods, such as the second half of an overly large meal (see page 52).

Why is it so hard to lose weight permanently?

Trying to lose weight and keep it off for good can feel like a battle you just can't win. And you can't escape the dieting advice. There are more weight-loss experts than you could shake a stick at. In health and lifestyle sections of magazines and newspapers few things take up more column inches than weight loss. You've tried diet after diet, but nothing sticks (except the pounds.)

Why, oh why can't you lose that excess weight? Frankly, it's because most of the experts doing most of the writing know about nutrition. But they know next to nothing about psychology. And if you already know what food is good for you, what's preventing you losing weight is likely to be difficulty with *how* you eat, not *what* you eat.

Here are three good reasons for struggling to lose weight, all of which are dealt with in this book.

1. Because you ignore what your body is telling you

If you've followed the rules of a diet that seems to work for other people, or exercised until you're blue (or red) in the face, and still the weight refuses to stay off, consider how much you've been listening to your body as you've tried to shift those pounds.

»   Have you noticed when you're hungry?

» Have you thought what to eat for breakfast on the basis of how many hours it will be before lunch?

No?

Then let me introduce you to your greatest friend and advisor for your weight-loss journey: your gut. More specifically, the connections between your gut and your brain. This book is all about using the signals from your gut to guide your eating.

When you engage your mind and tune into your gut when you are eating and whenever you think of eating, you'll have a reliable guide to when and how much to eat. Appetite Retraining shows you how to do this so that you can forget diet sheets and calorie counting and reach the weight you're comfortable with and stay there easily. Freedom around food, forever!

2. Because you try to change too much at once
» To lose weight you need to change your eating habits.
» To lose weight permanently you need to change your eating habits permanently.
» Changing habits is best done one step at a time.

This is why it is so ridiculously hard to lose weight following a conventional diet. Changing established habits takes effort and energy and is best done one step at a time. Conventional diets, on the other hand, require you to overhaul your eating habits overnight, which is near impossible to keep to.

But if you follow some simple steps to identify exactly what you need to change about your eating habits, and what you don't, you can achieve permanent weight loss without the Herculean effort of an athlete training for a marathon.

By choosing your favourite foods and learning how to eat in tune with your body, eating will be actually pleasurable while you lose the pounds.

And because you'll have established new eating habits, keeping the weight off will be easy.

'By setting yourself one manageable change at a time, you'll achieve success and boost your confidence.'

3. Because of mental blocks (saboteurs)

Self-sabotage doesn't happen for everyone. For some people, a clear plan of how to lose weight is enough. But if you've lost weight before, only to regain it and don't understand why, self-sabotage may be to blame. If you think this may be you, read on….

In the past, you've made a decision to lose weight and chosen what approach you're going to use. You start well. The enthusiasm of a fresh start with an approach that makes sense boosts your confidence and you're feeling optimistic.

But somehow, inexplicably, frustratingly and depressingly, a few weeks in, you find yourself doing exactly what you didn't want to do. Snacking when you didn't mean to, piling enough food onto your plate for two, or going back for seconds.

It feels as if you are two different people: the disciplined one who can keep on track and the devil-may-care one who can't be bothered with all the effort. And unfortunately the disciplined one seems to have quit.

The Appetite Retraining Programme helps you to identify your potential saboteurs or mental blocks. You'll understand how self-sabotage has derailed your weight loss efforts in the past and we'll tackle this head-on so that you don't have a repeat of the same old pattern.

Other factors that affect weight loss

Remember, we're all different. Even if you and a friend go on the same diet, or make the same single habit change using Appetite Retraining, your bodies will react differently. Your physical make-up, including your metabolism, how sensitive you are to insulin and other gut hormones, whether you have a medical condition such as an underactive thyroid, the composition of your gut biome (the billions of bacteria living in your gut) and whether you take medication, all affect how your body deals with the food you eat. If you're on medication and want to know whether what you're taking may make weight loss more difficult, speak to a pharmacist who can advise you whether to raise the issue with your doctor, or speak to your doctor in your next consultation.

Measuring your results

Even when you lose weight, be aware that it may not come off in the way you expect it to. When I started losing weight, the first three inches all came off my hip measurement and only when those three inches had been let go from my hips did I lose weight anywhere else. The habit change that produced the three-inch shrinkage was reducing my evening meal size. So, in my case, my body was holding on to three inches worth of fat on my hips because my dinner was too big.

Taking your starting chest, waist, hip and thigh measurements may be helpful in addition to weighing yourself, so that you can see what is changing. And if you want to influence your body shape as you go, you can talk to a qualified personal trainer about exercises that might help.

Weigh yourself as often as it helps. For many people this turns out to be daily, for others weekly and for some, not at all. This will depend on your experiences in the past of weighing yourself or being weighed. If being weighed has come to be associated with feeling publicly shamed, the scales may be associated with dread, and may not be a motivating influence at all. If, on the other hand, your competitive streak extends to competing with yourself, jumping on the scales may fire your commitment and focus. We're all different and nothing works for everyone.

Tracking your progress

On the next page is a blank graph for you to track your progress if you'd like to (you may prefer not to and that's fine too). There's a downloadable version of this graph on the Appetite Doctor® website – www.theappetitedoctor.co.uk.

In the left-hand column, write your current weight at the top of the 'Weight loss' column, next to the '0' and then go down in steps of a pound so that at the bottom the amount is 1 stone less than you weigh now.

Choose a particular day of the week to record your weight. If your chosen day is Friday, each Friday record your weight by placing a dot on the graph. It may help to write the actual dates of the Fridays along the bottom of the graph. Do the same on the Friday of week 2, 3, etc.

Joining the dots will give you a clear visual picture of how your weight loss is progressing. There are 14 weeks on the graph to give room for losing a pound a week on average, but if you get to a stone lighter sooner than 14 weeks, just start another graph with your new current weight at the top.

> **'You learned your current eating habits over a whole lifetime. You only need to change those that are causing the trouble, so don't clear out your pantry or fridge. This journey is about starting where you are now, and changing one unhelpful eating habit at a time.'**

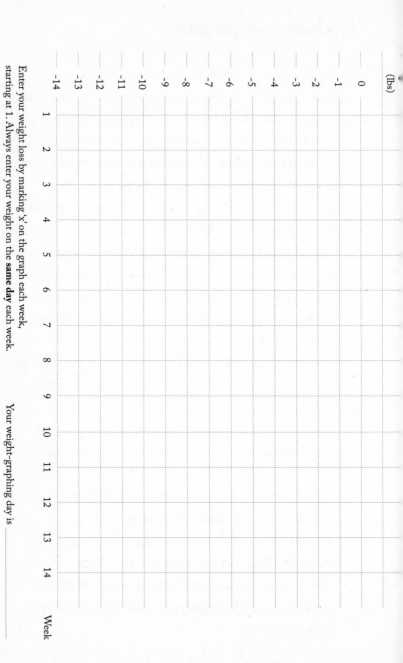

(lbs)

0
-1
-2
-3
-4
-5
-6
-7
-8
-9
-10
-11
-12
-13
-14

1 2 3 4 5 6 7 8 9 10 11 12 13 14 Week

Enter your weight loss by marking 'x' on the graph each week, starting at 1. Always enter your weight on the **same day** each week.

Your weight-graphing day is _____

Why maximizing pleasure matters

When it comes to weight loss and changing eating habits permanently, getting the most pleasure you can from eating is absolutely key. Because if we replace our old habit with something that is more delicious than before, it will be much easier to stick to.

Because of the way our brains evolved, we are hard-wired to move towards pleasure. We'll seek out foods that produce more pleasure. It's just part of our basic biology and psychology – an evolutionary thing.

And when we eat really delicious food when we're hungry, the feelings of hunger go away and we feel satisfied. What we've eaten really hits the spot. Eating like this (feel hungry, eat fabulous food, feel satisfied, stop eating) is a self-regulating system. But if you don't allow yourself to get hungry before eating, ordinary real food won't taste as good (because your taste buds weren't ready – see page 51). Instead you're more likely to ferret out something that has much higher levels of taste-bud stimulation.

How you eat has developed over the course of your whole lifetime. Your food likes and dislikes are the result of your genes, the foods your mother ate when you were in the womb, what she ate while breastfeeding you, your cultural background, your specific family food choices, and your own individual experiences of eating and the associations you've formed with particular foods. Maximizing pleasure involves keeping all of those foods you've come to love in your diet and probably discovering some new delicious ones.

Enhancing pleasure from food comes also from what we eat off. Professor Charles Spence, author of *Gastrophysics*, has studied how the crockery and cutlery we use influences how we taste food, and how satisfying the food is. Using heavier cutlery and crockery is a simple way to enhance our enjoyment of food.

The other way to increase your enjoyment of your food is to focus your attention on it as you eat. Mindfulness is hugely popular now, and eating each meal mindfully rather than distractedly makes a huge difference. Noticing the taste and texture of each mouthful, and the changing tastes you get from the food as you chew, allows you to get much more pleasure than if you eat quickly while doing something else.

'There's a certain amount of calories and pleasure available in every bite of food. You get the calories anyway when you eat, but you only get all the pleasure if you really focus on the taste.'

Outsmarting the experts

Food technologists have studied our pleasure responses to food to design ever-more delicious foods, but these 'hyper-palatable' foods come at a cost. Because the technologists have done such a thorough job researching our pleasure responses, they've created some we can't stop eating, such as Pringles.

If you weren't hungry when you started eating, you won't be able to use reducing hunger to gauge when to stop. Also, these engineered foods stimulate parts of the brain that cause you to keep eating, to a compulsive or addictive pattern instead of to the self-regulating system you used as a baby.

Appetite Retraining is the most delicious diet in the world because you eat the foods you have always loved and you may discover that you really love some new foods. And because you learn to wait to eat until you are definitely hungry, your taste buds are at their most sensitive.

There are no recipes in this book because you'll be cooking and eating the ones you've always loved. Appetite Retraining works whatever your culinary heritage. There's no need to look for obscure ingredients or clear out your pantry. There's no need for a huge blow-out meal before you start. With Appetite Retraining, how you eat tomorrow will be only slightly different from today and you won't make another change until that slightly different habit is easy to stick to.

Before we begin, it's worth understanding how your body's appetite system works. The more you tune in to it, the more you can use it to your advantage…

CHAPTER 2

—

The Appetite System

As we saw in Chapter 1, most diets focus solely on food. They are concerned with the types and quantity of food that will help get you to a particular end point. They provide rules or guidelines to follow, but they don't focus much, if at all, on what's happening inside your body. When I successfully lost a stone and a half with Weight Watchers 20 years ago (which I regained just six months later), I was overly hungry much of the time. I watched the clock until the next mealtime and struggled through on raw carrots and rice cakes – it was one point for three rice cakes if I remember rightly! I was continually battling against what my body was telling me. I was hungry and I needed to eat, but the rules meant that I couldn't afford to. If I used the points up too early, I'd be in total disarray by bedtime.

What you'll learn with Appetite Retraining is that it doesn't have to be like this – learning to recognize how hungry or full you are, and eating in tune with that, is the key to losing weight without putting a strain on your body. In the long run, as you settle in to a pattern of eating the right amount of food to keep you going until the next meal, perhaps with a snack to tide you over if needs be, you can learn to listen to your body's natural hunger and fullness signals and trust them to guide your eating. You will be in harmony with your body, and your body will respond well to that. There will be no more unbearable waiting while you struggle with feeling extremely hungry. You'll see how allowing yourself to get definitely, but not overly, hungry by each meal allows you to lose weight. And by stopping eating each meal when you're just full – not stuffed – means you'll definitely be hungry by the next meal.

The way that your body and brain regulates eating is mind-bogglingly complex. It is governed by two systems: the system that deals with self-regulation (homeostasis), which is controlled from the hypothalamus, and the system that deals with pleasure and pain – which is controlled by the limbic system (see page 56).

Even having just a rudimentary understanding of what's going on inside your body and brain can help you think about how to eat and how to work with your biology and psychology, not against them.

'When you follow a diet that puts you out of touch with your body and brain, you're under pressure from the word go.'

How we've lost our way with food

Over recent decades, the way we eat has become increasingly divorced from the way the human body evolved. Over millions of years, our digestive system evolved to allow us to eat a meal that gives us enough energy for a few hours. Once that meal is used up, signals from our gut and other organs tell our brain that it is time to eat again. We experience these signals as hunger. When we eat, the hunger signals are switched off and we start to register feelings of increasing fullness and we have the energy we need for the next few hours.

Our brains evolved to seek out food and respond to the sight or smell of it by salivating, so that our body is ready to digest it. Finding food took time and effort and preparing it for eating was demanding work. But food is no longer scarce in much of the developed world – in fact, it's available ready-to-eat, just about everywhere and often round-the-clock. In this new environment of plentiful and often cheap food, many of us are confused about what to eat. This is true even for people who are highly competent, successful and intelligent. I've worked with doctors who understand the workings of the human body better than anyone, and are aware of the damage that overeating causes to the body, but who feel bemused and embarrassed that they themselves can't always control their own eating.

Your gut and how it works

Humans have a stomach that is about the size of a fist, which is supplied with food by the oesophagus – a muscular pipe that moves food from the mouth after swallowing. After passing through the stomach, food enters the small intestine (ileum) and from there the large intestine (colon). These two parts of the intestine make up a muscular tube several metres in length in which nutrients and water are absorbed into the body. Once food has completed its journey through the intestine, anything left enters the rectum and is expelled into the toilet as poo.

This structure and function of the gut, from mouth to anus, means that we're adapted to eat meals with gaps between them. How long those gaps are depends on the size of our meals, and what foods we consume. We are not cows. We do not have to graze continually to supply our bodies with the nutrients and energy needed for life. And we are not snakes – we can't ingest an enormous meal and spend days digesting it. If we do start to eat like cows or snakes, we are likely to pile weight on.

A key biological process swings into action once the food from your last meal has finished digesting. Your body switches from digestion to repairing damaged cells, and to cleaning your gut. In that gap between meals when you're beginning to feel hungry, your body is putting its house in order.

Two particular features of how the gut works are key to Appetite Retraining.

1. The stomach is like a pouch with a valve at its entry point from the oesophagus (the cardiac sphincter) and another valve at its exit point into the duodenum (the pyloric sphincter). It's made of muscle and as food pours in, the stomach wall expands. Specialized nerve cells in the wall of the stomach (mechanoreceptors) are activated when this stretching occurs and they send messages to the brain to say that food is entering the stomach. They register the volume of food you've eaten. Because these are nerve cell (neuronal) transmissions, they are super-fast like high-speed broadband.

2. The small intestine and large intestine are where absorption of food takes place. Gut hormones, such as leptin, help to break down food and send signals to the brain about the food that is being digested. They register the metabolites (constituent products of the breakdown) of what you've just eaten. Hormonal signals are chemical (not neuronal) and these travel via the bloodstream. The speed of these signals is much slower than the signals from the mechanoreceptors in the stomach wall. More snail-mail than fibre optics. It takes upwards of 20 minutes for the hormonal information from the gut to register with different brain centres.

Both the immediate neuronal messages from the stomach and the slower hormonal messages from the intestine are part of our Appetite System's way of telling the brain that we can stop eating as we've had enough food.

> **'We have two types of signals telling our brain about hunger and fullness levels: fast neuronal signals from the stomach and slow hormonal signals from the intestine. We need to tune in to those fast signals to help prevent us overeating.'**

How hunger and fullness work

We experience these messages (neuronal from the stomach and hormonal from the intestine) as a sense of increasing fullness, and it is the immediate neuronal signals from your stomach that you need to re-learn to listen to, in order to gauge how much you've eaten.

Because the mechanism is due to the stomach wall stretching, this is all about the volume, not content of what you've eaten. So the same volume of steamed broccoli is registered as the same volume of French fries or ice cream or lasagne.

If you ignore the immediate signals being registered from the mechanoreceptors in your stomach wall, you'll have to rely on the hormonal signals from your intestine. But, as we've seen, these take 20 minutes or so to fully register, and you can consume an awful lot of food in those 20 minutes.

Think of Christmas dinner: that celebratory meal can involve serious over-catering, but you don't feel completely stuffed and slightly drugged until after you've polished off seconds of Christmas pudding, by which time you're groaning and full of regret, and you fall asleep in front of the TV. If you were a snake, this wouldn't matter and you'd hide under a log for a day or two until you'd digested it all. But being human, on Boxing Day morning your internal clock (see below) is telling you it's time to eat, and you're off again.

When you learn to listen to the fullness signals from your stomach, you can retrain yourself around portion sizes, so that you eat what your body needs for the next few hours. In the time following your last meal, your body is at work digesting and absorbing the goodness (or otherwise) from the food. The phenomenally complex system that governs this extracts different elements from the food (glucose, fatty acids, amino acids, vitamins etc) and gut hormones send messages to the brain about how far the process of using up the last meal has progressed. As nutrients are transported to where they are needed or where they are going to be stored, hormones (including ghrelin) signal that the food from the last meal has now been used up and your body has to switch to using up its energy reserves.

These signals are experienced as increasing hunger and they only begin once we switch over to using up stored energy. That stored energy is fat, so those signals tell us that we are now burning a bit of stored fat. BINGO! That's exactly what we want in order to lose weight. Appetite Retraining teaches you to use those signals of increasing hunger to guide when to start eating, and to tolerate feelings of mild hunger so that you wait to eat until you are definitely hungry. In that space between mild and definite hunger, you will burn a bit of fat. (It's not this simple in reality, but this is the gist of what happens as you get hungry.) By burning this fat, your body has been given a new bit of energy so the hunger signals are switched off again. This pattern of switching off hunger signals because a bit of fat has been burned for energy means that tolerating mild hunger comes in phases – it's not continuous. In a while – maybe 15 minutes, maybe half an hour – you'll begin noticing sensations of hunger starting up again. And they will get stronger each time they're triggered, and it's your job to notice when these sensations are definite hunger as opposed to slight hunger. To enable your body to burn a little stored fat before each meal.

If waiting to eat until you're definitely hungry makes you feel uneasy or anxious, don't worry. That is entirely normal and is covered in Chapter 7.

The purpose of feeling hungry is to orient us away from other things and towards seeking out food. It's a basic part of how our Appetite System works to keep us alive and healthy by getting us to eat. The next part of this system we'll look at is the role our taste buds play.

Your taste buds

Your taste buds are receptor cells in the mouth and nose, which detect certain qualities of food and drink. These are salt, sweet, bitter, umami and sour. Combinations of these give rise to flavour and, together with other qualities of food, such as fat content, produce the overall level of palatability of the food.

When our taste buds are more sensitive, we experience more flavour – and they are at their most sensitive when we are hungry. This is why the Ancient Greeks described hunger as 'the best seasoning'. So a particular food eaten when you're hungry tastes much better than the same food eaten when you're not, and when you increase the amount of pleasure you get from eating, your appetite is more satisfied.

Part of the system that helps us know when to stop eating is taste-specific satiety – our taste buds become less sensitive to the food we are eating, bite by bite. The first few bites of any dish are the most tasty, but if we then switch to a different food, that new taste hasn't been desensitized to the same degree, so we're likely to enjoy that more than we would if we continued eating more of the first food. This is why pudding may be alluring, even though you've had your fill of your main course and why the babies I mentioned in Chapter 1 (see page 23) are interested in the dessert when they've rejected any more main course.

Your nose

You'll be very familiar with the way that the smell of baking bread or fresh coffee activates your appetite. Your mouth may be watering now just reading those words. We're born with an automatic reaction ('unconditioned response') of salivating in response to food, just like Pavlov's famous dogs (see page 191). Because the volatile compounds in food are detected by our noses, we learn to expect food when we smell it – and when we expect food, our appetite system kicks in to action whether we're hungry or not.

Your eyes

The sight of food itself is enough to activate our digestive juices and sharpen our appetite. When you catch sight of a food that you know you love, your memories of the pleasure of eating it are triggered, and you are more likely to seek it out without even realizing it. This is a sub-conscious process and happens even if the sight of the food is too quick (subliminal) to be registered consciously.

The lure of food
The sight of food we love activates our desire to eat it, and advertisers and supermarkets know this – that's why they use visual images of food to get us to buy more. Later in the book, I'll explain how to deal with the visual triggering of your appetite, so that you can stop yourself eating just because you've caught sight of a cake advert out of the corner of your eye, or had a fleeting image of the 'golden arches' M as you speed along the road.

Your mouth

As we begin to chew and taste our food, the process of digestion begins and it's where we hope to detect danger in the food. If something is poisonous, or the food has gone off, our sense of taste may pick that up and force us to spit it out. How we chew food influences how much taste and pleasure we get from it, and we'll return to this point in the section on Maximizing Pleasure from food in Chapter 9.

Your brain

Your brain has a massive part to play in Appetite Retraining. After all, it was probably listening to what your brain told you to eat rather than what your gut was trying to tell you that led you to gain weight in the first place. We are going to note a few key brain areas and functions that are relevant to Appetite Retraining here, so that you have reference points when we come to these later in the book.

1. The hypothalamus

This thermostat-like centre helps us regulate our basic bodily functions to allow us to maintain a state of equilibrium (homeostasis). When these functions, such as blood glucose level, temperature and hydration, move out of the comfortable range, bodily and mental systems are set in motion to restore harmony. For example, if your temperature is rising, your pores will open and sweating will help to cool you. If the temperature continues to rise, signals to your conscious brain tell it to take action to cool down by, for example, opening a window or taking off a sweater. Eating is partly regulated by the hypothalamus, which is helpful to keep our eating regulated and our weight constant. However, it's also strongly influenced by two other systems: the pleasure system and the anxiety system.

2. The pleasure system and hedonic overeating

The areas of the brain (the cortico-limbic structures) involved in processing pleasure are involved in the anticipation of eating and particularly in eating certain types of food. Your favourite treats are at the top of this list, so now we're in the realm not just of satisfying the body's need for sustenance, but the brain's desire for stimulation of its pleasure centres. The big food corporations are ahead of us here as they have worked out what particular flavour and texture combinations, in what sequence, push our pleasure buttons most exquisitely, by releasing a cascade of flavours and textures that blow us away. Those foods are manufactured to be what Dr David Kessler calls 'hyper-palatable'. The pleasure centres are governed by positive feedback loops that trigger us to desire more as we eat, not less. This system reacts to the amount of reward rather than the amount of energy in the food, and each time we experience pleasure, our brain stores the information under 'things to do again, and soon!'

We'll look at how to include these foods in the overall range of what you eat, without allowing them to overwhelm your pleasure system so that you are unable to stop eating them. You probably have no problem stopping eating your favourite vegetable, but your favourite treat? That's another story. Not everyone develops cravings, because we all have different levels of response to pleasurable cues. If you're someone who does struggle to resist overeating certain foods, see pages 198–200 for advice on how to reduce cravings.

3. The limbic system: anxiety, stress and emotional eating

Anxiety and fear are the body's way of helping us deal with danger. The brain centre that is involved in detecting such threats is the amygdala, part of the limbic system. When a threat is detected, the amygdala triggers the release of adrenaline from the adrenal glands to help deal with the danger. In this 'fight or flight' state, our heart rate surges to pump oxygen to our muscles.

Extreme hunger is, of course, dangerous, and will trigger the fear response, but many of us with plenty to eat have developed a fear of even mild hunger, which is not at all dangerous. If you have become anxious about feeling hungry, established techniques for overcoming learned fears will help you (see pages 211–215).

Stress affects people differently. Some of us eat more when we are stressed and some of us go off our food. Eating more when you're experiencing a stressful event appears to be related to your background levels of chronic stress, and your biological make-up. Stress affects the areas of the brain that deal with reward, and chronic stress heightens the sensitivity of the reward centre, resulting in increased appetitive drive. Learning about stress and how to reduce it is covered in Chapter 8.

Your internal clock

We have a number of internal 'clocks' that keep time over each 24-hour cycle, in tune with the earth's rotation. Night and day produce different levels of light, and our bodies adapt to the light/dark cycle of where we live. If we move rapidly between one daily cycle and another by flying East or West, the resulting jet lag is the consequence of external triggers being out of synch with our internal clocks.

Our appetite-regulating hormones follow a 24-hour pattern, and we come to associate certain times of day or night with eating. These time-triggers are quite powerful for many of us, and you may be aware of itching to eat at around 12.30 pm if that's when you're used to having lunch, because your appetite system is swinging in to action in line with what your internal clocks are saying.

Having regular times to eat works in tune with your body's daily appetite cycle and we'll talk more about establishing an eating routine that fits around your lifestyle and works in tune with your body in Chapter 5.

Listening to your gut

As we've seen, the digestive system and brain are at work guiding our eating and appetite. We need to use both together, but modern super-stimulating foods, available round the clock cheaply and in abundance, mean that it's easy to rely more on your brain than your gut. Too much brain focus is not a good thing if it means ignoring your gut.

When we ignore or override our natural internal hunger and fullness signals, we eat in response to external triggers. We're more likely to eat things we see and eat beyond the point of being full. Because we have memories of super-pleasurable foods, those will be the ones we reach for, particularly at times of stress or anxiety. We're likely to eat until the plate is empty instead of stopping when we're just full. We're not likely to get much pleasure from the food as our taste buds won't be so sensitive if we're not hungry, and because we won't be eating what we have a real appetite for, but what our brain remembers was really pleasurable before.

If we tune in to what our gut is saying, we can gauge when to eat and when to stop. As we've seen, we digest and store the nutrients and energy from our last meal and, as we do so, our gut and other organs send increasingly strong signals to our brain to get us to eat again. As we eat, our stomach wall receptor cells and intestinal hormones send signals to our brain to tell us we've had enough. The meal we've eaten will be enough to keep us going for a certain amount of time, depending on how much and what we ate.

The Appetite Pendulum™

The cyclical pattern of eating and (mini-) fasting suits our biology and means that we don't have to eat constantly. It's like a pendulum. My Appetite Pendulum™ (see below) gives you a way of thinking about your level of hunger or fullness at any point – it is a key part of the Appetite Retraining Programme.

On pages 90–92 and pages 188–190, I explain how to use the Appetite Pendulum™, but for now just see whether you can gauge where you are on the Appetite Pendulum™ below right now. The extremes of the scale refer to feeling completely stuffed at one end (+5), which is how you'd feel about half an hour after a very large meal. At the other end (–5), you're likely to feel strong sensations in your stomach, perhaps growling or rumbling – this is how you feel when you have missed a meal and it's now many hours since you ate.

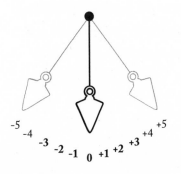

+5 uncomfortably full
+4 very full
+3 just full
+2 nearly full
+1 not sure, probably not hungry
 0 neutral
-1 not sure, probably a bit hungry
-2 slightly hungry
-3 definitely hungry
-4 very hungry
-5 extremely hungry

What if you can't detect feelings of hunger or fullness?

To begin with, some people find it hard to gauge their hunger or fullness levels. If you're struggling to work out where you are on the Appetite Pendulum™, I'll show you how to use meal-size reduction strategies, while you gradually learn to listen to the hunger and fullness signals from your gut. That means judging how much you need by looking, so you can still lose weight by training your eye to judge what amounts lead to weight loss and then to maintaining your goal weight.

Appetite Retraining is all about learning to eat in tune with your natural hunger and fullness signals. Rather than attempt to do this all at once, we'll take things one step at a time, partly so that it's not too much strain on your system to make the change, and partly so that each step becomes easy and automatic – a habit, in other words. And it's the fact that you'll form new eating habits that makes the weight loss you achieve easy to sustain.

In the next chapter we'll look at the psychology of eating habits. I'll explain why we form habits in the first place and what's needed to change an established habit.

Mo had always been very active and after a sporting injury curtailed the amount of physical activity he could do, he found himself eating more and gaining weight. He hadn't had a problem with his weight before, but he started to feel self-conscious around his sporty friends. He was keen to return to eating less, but was worried that if he did, he would be hungry all the time and would start overeating again. I explained the way that hunger signals work (see pages 49–51), and that when we get hungry it is our body telling us that we're having to switch to fat burning. Mo was particularly interested in the fact that when this happens, the hunger signals are switched off for a while, so the feelings of hunger come and go. This gave him the confidence to tolerate mild feelings of hunger and start losing weight.

CHAPTER 3

—

The Psychology of Eating and Appetite

As we saw in Chapter 1, most diets require you to change completely how you eat overnight, which puts phenomenal pressure on you psychologically. We're not built to make dramatic changes suddenly. It's not how our evolutionary psychology works. In this chapter I'll show you what simple features of our very complex psychology can help us with weight loss. The first thing to understand is that we have two systems involved in learning and memory, which dictate what happens when we try to change how we eat, whether we realize it or not.

One system in the brain has a very small capacity. It takes very high levels of energy and deals with what is happening to us right now. It's concerned with processing or digesting the information coming in, and attending to anything new we need to learn. This is called Working Memory. The other system has enormous capacity. It's like a filing system, which contains the information we already know – facts, faces, names and dates, our life story and the words to songs from the pop charts from our teenage years. This is long-term memory and it includes established habit sequences.

These two systems work co-operatively so that anything that we don't need to be focusing on is transferred out of the small Working Memory to the long-term store. And if we need to access stored information, we can get hold of it, except stuff that we didn't store properly in the first place, such as what we did with the house keys when we came in! As we'll see in this chapter, it's essential to have enough space in your Working Memory to focus on developing new eating habits.

What is a habit?

A habit is a pattern that has become so familiar that you do it on autopilot – like brushing your teeth. Once upon a time someone taught you how to brush your teeth. In the years since, you will have given it little or no thought despite doing it a couple of times a day.

Habits save us huge amounts of mental effort for tasks that we do over and again. When we see our toothbrush by the sink, there's no need to think about what to do with it. Our hand and subconscious brain put in motion the sequence of

open toothpaste

˅

squeeze on to brush

˅

start brushing

A habit is formed when you follow the same sequence repeatedly. It's thanks to the brain relegating a familiar pattern to subconscious, automatic control, so a habit is an automated action sequence, where the whole sequence follows automatically when the start of it is triggered.

When you perform an action for the first time, you use conscious thought and deliberate intention. Your brain registers a memory trace. If you do the same thing again quite soon, the memory is re-traced and becomes stronger. Keep practising the same thing and you need less and less

Working Memory as the sequence is established in your long-term memory.

What characterizes a habit is that as soon as you see a trigger (the toothbrush by the sink), the whole sequence plays out without you even thinking about it. Except if something in the sequence is out of order, like the toothpaste tube being empty. Then your brain reverts to using Working Memory to sort out the glitch, before setting you back on the habit sequence.

This is a brilliant system. It helped us create the wonders of the world and walk on the moon. If NASA scientists had to re-think tooth-brushing every morning, there's no way Apollo 11 would have made it off the launch pad.

There is a downside, of course, and that is what keeps you eating too much ice cream when you promised yourself faithfully yesterday that you wouldn't.

'Keep practising the same thing and you need less and less Working Memory as the sequence is established in your long-term memory.'

How to change an established habit

In order to change a habit, you have to get it out of the automated sequence and bring it under conscious control, just until you've replaced it with a new habit. This means bringing it into Working Memory.

Working Memory is the name for the workspace in our brain that deals with what's happening right now. It has lots of feeds into it, but a very small capacity. It's a high-energy operation with a narrow focus on what's going on at the present time, but it can switch between different information inputs rapidly. Different people have different Working Memory capacity, so some of us can hold more in mind or are better able to deal with complex problems.

As I said, to move from an existing to a new habit, we've got to bring the old habit into Working Memory in order to create a new action sequence by doing the new, desired habit repeatedly until it becomes automatic and is then itself a habit, relegated to automatic control.

bring current unhelpful habit into Working Memory

⌄

consciously change unhelpful habit within Working Memory

⌄

repeat new habit until it becomes automatic and a part
of long-term memory

Consider an example of how this relates to everyday life, not to do with eating. When something you do very regularly changes, such as how you travel to work or which school your child goes to, you're so used to the old pattern that if you don't consciously think about where you're going (i.e. bringing the route into Working Memory), you'll get the wrong bus, go to the old workplace or turn up at the wrong school.

Another example is if you are used to driving a British right-hand drive car on British roads and then hire a left-hand drive car and start driving on the continent. The controls are the wrong way round and you're on the wrong side of the road, so you can no longer rely on your brain's autopilot to drive safely. You have to concentrate on each manoeuvre and think deliberately about what you're doing. Roundabouts are a hazard, as are left turns. And woe betide anyone who tries to ask you a question when you set off from the car hire depot, with your brain in overload. But after a fortnight you'll be whizzing around like a local, because your brain will have re-sequenced your driving skills. What has happened during the holiday is that you've used your Working Memory to perform the new driving actions, and each time you've repeated them, you've strengthened the sequence more and more, so that by the end you are no longer having to use any Working Memory to drive other than when you come upon something unexpected, just like you've always done on UK roads.

The same thing is true of unhelpful eating habits. To change a habit you need to get the automatic action sequence back in to conscious awareness (Working Memory), and replace it with performing a different sequence. To do this, you need to work out what that new sequence will be, step by step. You'll need to keep repeating the new sequence over and again until it becomes the new habit, at which point you won't need to think about it so much. It will have become what you automatically do, and at that point it will be easier to do the new thing than the old one.

Let's look at how this might work if you want to stop eating biscuits with your mid-morning coffee. The old automatic sequence is something like

put kettle on

˅

put coffee in cup

˅

go to biscuit tin

˅

take out biscuits

˅

add hot water to coffee

˅

go and sit down, eat and drink both together

To change this habit, you need to get this automatic sequence in to conscious Working Memory. This requires a bit of advanced planning to nudge yourself into conscious thinking when coffee time arrives. You could put a note to yourself on the coffee jar or the kettle and move the biscuit tin somewhere else so that you'd have to think about where it is, which gives you time to remember that you're not planning to have the biscuits. You could sit somewhere different to have your coffee. And you'd be wise to put something new and nice instead of the biscuits in to the sequence such as having a book or magazine to read. If you are hungry you could have a favourite piece of fruit ready and waiting where the biscuits used to be, or a note to remind you that your favourite snack is in the fridge. So the sequence becomes:

put kettle on and notice the reminder

˅

put coffee in cup

˅

get your magazine/book/fruit out

˅

add hot water to coffee

˅

go and sit in new place and enjoy your coffee with something to read or the new type of snack

Why is it hard to change an existing habit?

There are very good reasons why habit change isn't easy and by knowing what these are, you can find ways to work round them.

1. You don't know what you're trying to change
Put simply, habit change is hard when you're shooting in the dark and don't really know what you're meant to be doing. So having a clear step-by-step plan for your new eating habit is a must.

2. You don't really know why you're doing it
You are doing it to achieve a goal, but if your goal is vague or woolly, it's more likely that you'll lose your way. We'll talk more about this in Chapter 6 when we look at strengthening motivation.

3. You haven't got enough available bandwidth in your Working Memory
If your Working Memory is already overloaded, trying to add something to its workload is going to fail. Just like your phone when its storage is full and whatever you do, it refuses to take a photo of that cute kitten you desperately want to post on Instagram. Remember that your Working Memory capacity is very limited, so to change an established habit you'll need

some spare bandwidth to be able to succeed. What this means in practice is that if you're going through a tough time and have a lot on your mind, by all means read on and learn about what you can do when the time is right, but don't start trying to make changes now. It will only add to your feelings of failure.

4. You haven't got the energy needed
As well as sufficient bandwidth, you need your Working Memory to have enough energy to function. When you don't charge your phone, however much space it has free, it's not going to send that text. And if you're low on energy, because you haven't slept or are continually drained by the demands on you, your Working Memory is going to be like a phone with a flat battery. Not able to do much.

Now we are going to look at which habits you need to change, and how to do that. I'll talk you through how to give your Working Memory a fighting chance of forming the new habits, dealing with likely hurdles as you go.

'Eating isn't like smoking or biting your nails. It's essential to life, so you can't simply quit.'

Work out if and why you want to lose weight

Your first task is to ask yourself, 'Do I really want to do this?' To answer this, ask yourself the following four questions:

1. What will my best benefit be?

For example, you might benefit most by improving your health, appearance or self-confidence. This is a really valuable thing to get straight at the outset, because this is what you're going to be relying on to get you through any hiccups and any temptation to give up. Which might well happen at some point. The following three short visualization exercises will help you work out your best benefit. Once you know that, you'll use that as and when you need it throughout the rest of the book.

Best benefit 1: Looking good

Bring to mind how you will look when you have reached your goal weight. Think of a particular outfit you have that would look better at that weight. Alternatively, imagine yourself in something you would buy if you were slimmer. Picture yourself in front of a full-length mirror wearing these clothes. Set the lighting in your imagination to show this outfit off to its best effect. If it is an evening outfit, have warm lighting as if it is dark outside. If it is a daytime outfit, imagine how much sunshine you would like to be flooding into the room and how you would like it to fall on you so that you look your best. Really tune in to how nice that feels. Notice where the feelings are in your body and focus on them. Turn around in front of the mirror and see how you look from all angles. Choose the feature you will most look forward to focusing on.

Best benefit 2: Feeling fit and healthy

Bring to mind how you will feel physically when you have reached your goal weight. Think of a particular activity that will be easier or feel better at that weight – perhaps walking, cycling or dancing. We'll use the example of walking for this illustration. Imagine yourself walking in your favourite place. Notice your surroundings and choose a time of day and weather you like best. Tune in to how it feels for your body to be moving freely and easily. Notice the contact of your feet with the earth on each step. Be aware of feeling alive in your body. Really tune in to how good that feels. Notice where the feelings of health and fitness are in your body and focus on them.

Best benefit 3: Feeling confident

Bring to mind how you will feel in yourself when you have reached your goal weight. Think of a particular situation in which you'll feel more confident at that weight. It might be with a particular person, or in a group. Notice how it feels to be in your body at this new weight. Notice your confident posture and your confident expression – smiling, calm or serious – whatever will feel best to you. Tune in to what this feels like in your body – grounded and calm. Notice the thoughts that are in your mind – positive and focused on the situation in hand. Really tune in to how nice that feels. Notice where the feelings of confidence are in your body and focus on them.

Now you've tried all three, choose the visualization that gives you the strongest positive feeling. There are two uses for this: one is to do this visualization daily to strengthen your connection to your goal, and the other is to bring your best benefit to mind whenever you feel your motivation flagging.

2. What will life really be like when I lose weight?
Alongside being clear about what you'll gain, it's useful to recognize what you'll lose. Change involves both gaining something and losing something else. The first part of change involves loss. You will probably have got used to being the weight you are now, even if you don't like it, so the next questions to get clear in your mind are:

» Does it feel safe for me to lose weight permanently? You might be concerned that people will envy you, that important relationships will be negatively affected or that you might have to deal with attractiveness and intimacy.
» Do I deserve to lose weight permanently?
» Will I still feel like me if I lose weight permanently?

As you can see, these questions all relate to what you might lose apart from the inches. You might lose the ability to avoid envy, or hide from intimacy. Your sense of yourself is likely to change towards feeling able to deserve good things, if you don't already. We'll return to these issues later on, in the section on self-belief (see pages 169–175).

3. What won't change when I lose weight?

The other side of anticipating what will change when you reach your goal is realizing what won't. When you pin your hopes on a particular goal, you can lose sight of the limitations of achieving it. As Shauna Reid who describes her own success with weight loss says in *The Amazing Adventures of Diet Girl*:

'You know what's funny about losing a stack of weight? Nothing really changes. All that happens is that you lose the thing upon which you used to hang all your neuroses. Fat has shape and substance; you can poke it with a stick. It's a scapegoat and a handy excuse. Once you start to lose it, you realize you're stuck with the same neurotic core.'

This doesn't mean giving up your goals. Just being clear about what they are and what they will and won't give you.

4. Is this the right time to lose weight?

There will be times in your life when focusing on losing weight would be particularly difficult, because of other major things happening. As I explained at the beginning of this chapter (see page 65), you need space in your Working Memory to focus on changing habits. So, if you are struggling to function reasonably well day to day, losing weight may be a step too far right now. You can still read this book now and get a feel for what you will do when you are ready, and maybe set yourself reminders in the months ahead to check in with whether it's a good time to start. On the other hand, life is rarely smooth, and putting off losing weight could leave it permanently postponed. So, if despite other things going on, you are coping reasonably well day to day, starting now is realistic. In Chapter 8 we'll deal with 'emotional eating', which will show you how to deal with difficult feelings without turning to food. Which means that you'll be able to deal with the normal ups and downs of life without excess eating.

Now you've looked at the four questions, you'll know whether you really do want to lose weight now. If you've realized that you're not sure, or not ready, you can still read on and get a feel for what it will involve when you are ready, but you won't need to go through a doomed attempt at weight loss. You can instead wait until you're at a point where the four questions have different answers and you're ready to go.

'Daily visualization of your best benefit will strengthen your connection to your goal. Bringing your best benefit to mind also helps boost your motivation when it is flagging.'

Keep good eating habits and let go of unhelpful ones

Good eating habits fuel and nourish your body and mind, but when you look to food to do more than this, for example by treating it as a hobby, or by using it as medication or as a comfort or a distraction, you consume too much. And because of human biology, when you swallow food, your body breaks it down and stores what's not needed as fat. We evolved like this during times of food shortages, and the fat stores were used for energy when food then became scarce. Your body can't tell that the cake you've just eaten wasn't needed. It doesn't have one system for food we need and one for food we don't. It treats all food the same.

Too much food on offer
What constitutes a helpful eating habit depends on where you are. If food is really scarce, it is a good idea to eat what's available whenever it is available, but that's not true of the Western world. If, like most people, you live in a home with a well-stocked fridge and cupboards, eating what's available whenever it is available is a recipe for disaster.

Which habits do you need to change?

The habits you need to change are personal to you – they are the ones that are keeping you heavier than you want to be: eating beyond the point of being just full and eating when you're not hungry. It's important to remember that you should only change what you need to change. If it's not broke, don't fix it. We're going to look at making changes one step at a time, leaving everything that's OK as it is and changing what's not. To start with, we'll identify the particular things you need to change. Here's a list of the most common unhelpful eating habits – tick those that apply to you.

Hannah worked in an office with people who regularly brought in tempting home-made bakes. Her sweet tooth led to a pattern of grazing on cake and biscuits during the morning, then not needing lunch. By the time she got home she was very hungry and had a large meal with dessert and wine, which she really enjoyed with her husband. She didn't tend to snack after dinner, unless she was feeling upset or stressed, and then found herself eating sweet foods. On the Unhelpful Eating Habits checklist Hannah ticked: My portion sizes are too big/I eat dessert even if I'm already full/I eat something just because it's there/I eat when I'm bored/ stressed/agitated/anxious although I'm not hungry/I eat too much unhealthy food. (See page 83 for the habits Hannah worked on.)

Unhelpful Eating Habits Checklist

1.   **Eating too much at any one time**

☐   My portion sizes are too big

☐   I eat dessert even if I'm already full

☐   I have times when I binge on unhealthy foods and can't stop

2.   **Problems with your eating routine**

☐   My eating routine is erratic or non-existent

☐   I skip meals quite often to save calories

3.   **Eating when you're not hungry**

☐   I eat out of habit (e.g. I have biscuits with tea)

☐   I eat something just because it's there

☐   I eat extra food now in case I'm hungry later

☐   I get cravings for particular foods and tend to give in to them whether I'm hungry or not

☐   I eat when I feel bored/stressed/angry/agitated/anxious, even though I'm not hungry

4.   **Problems with what you're eating**

☐   I find that food I expect to enjoy isn't satisfying so I keep trying other foods

☐   I have an unbalanced diet

☐   I eat too much unhealthy food

Each of these types of habits is dealt with in this book.

Your next step

Look back at what you ticked on the Unhelpful Eating Habits Checklist. Choose up to four habits that you want to change and put them on the list below. If you've ticked more than four, just choose the ones you think will be most important to change. Once you've made the first steps, you can look again at what else to work on.

These will be the first four steps on your journey to permanent weight loss. If there are fewer than four, that's no problem.

1. _____

2. _____

3. _____

4. _____

For Hannah, there were three habits we agreed to work on:

1. Stop eating cake and biscuits at work just because they are there (by introducing a delicious sustaining breakfast of avocado on toast – one of Hannah's favourite foods) and stopping this Opportunistic Eating (see Chapter 7).

2. Reduce evening meal size (see Chapter 4).

3. Stop emotional eating (see Chapter 8).

» For items to do with stopping eating when you're just full, see Chapter 4.
» If you have either of the 'Problems with eating routine' items on your list, see Chapter 5.
» For items to do with waiting to eat until you're definitely hungry, see Chapter 7.
» For emotional eating, see Chapter 8.
» For items to do with what you eat, see Chapter 9.

CHAPTER 4

—

Stop Eating When You're Full

If you eat more than you need to regularly, you will gain weight and keep it on. Fact. Learning how to stop eating when you're just full is one of the most important parts of Appetite Retraining because eating just enough of a meal is the only way you can get definitely hungry by the next meal. And, remember, it's when you start to feel hungry between meals that your body actually burns stored fat (see page 50).

To stop eating when you're just full, you need to tune in to the immediate signals from your stomach to your brain registering how much volume of food has entered your stomach. With Appetite Retraining you keep the amount of food consistent across meals. The same volume of porridge stretches your stomach to the same degree as that volume of green beans or ice cream or sausages. And it's the amount that gets you to feel just full (+3 on the Appetite Pendulum™) that you learn to *see* as your new normal meal size.

You choose what types of foods to eat based on how long it will be until the next meal – for example, porridge or sausages will keep you going for longer than green beans or ice cream. People often tell me that they try to avoid feeling hungry by piling their plate up with 'healthy' foods by which they usually mean vegetables. That is an alternative way to eat, and may help you lose weight, but it's not helpful for Appetite Retraining because a pile of vegetables will keep you in a pattern of getting overly full and still fearful of mild hunger.

Having a small meal of just vegetables is likely to mean you'll be hungry again quite soon. As you'll see later in the book, there are times when that's exactly what you need.

This chapter deals with the three Unhelpful Eating Habits which involve eating beyond the point of being just full.

1. You regularly eat meals that are too large

Many of us eat too much either because we're enjoying the food and don't want to stop, or we're eating mindlessly and not paying attention. Either way, if your portion sizes are too big, regularly, you're constantly putting more food into your body than it can use. Whatever that food is, healthy or not, excess food will be converted into fat. And your body will store it in your fat cells. To lose weight, your body needs to be able to start releasing those fat stores. It will do that whenever you've run out of energy from the last meal you ate, so a hugely important part of Appetite Retraining is altering the size of each meal, so that you'll have most of the energy you need for a few hours in that meal, but not quite enough so that your body will switch to burning a bit of stored fat before your next meal.

2. You eat dessert even though you're already full

If you have a sweet tooth, perhaps desserts are your downfall – but they don't need to be. You can still have your favourite puddings and sweets once you learn how to judge how much to eat, and to gauge when you really want that sweet food. In this chapter I'll explain how eating desserts or sweets fits in to Appetite Retraining

3. You binge eat

Overeating to the extent that you feel out of control is more common than you might think. It is thought that about 12 million people in the UK suffer from compulsive overeating to some extent. This includes people who feel they binge occasionally through to people who suffer with an eating disorder such as Binge Eating Disorder (see page 109).

Jack didn't really enjoy his job and looked forward to the evening, when he would wind down with his partner over dinner and a bottle of wine. After the main course, Jack enjoyed cheese and biscuits with another glass of wine. Once the dishes were cleared away, he often fell asleep in front of the TV. He'd thought about changing his job, but never seemed to have any energy or free time to do anything about it.

On the Unhelpful Eating Habits checklist Jack ticked 'My portion sizes are too big' and 'I eat dessert even if I'm already full' – his 'dessert' was the cheese and biscuits. Although he enjoyed winding down over a good meal, he didn't like feeling bloated most nights, and falling asleep in front of the TV meant he was missing out on doing more interesting activities, and on the opportunity to look online for a new job. He also wanted to stop gaining weight. He chose to work on reducing his evening meal size and not eating cheese and biscuits as a regular 'dessert'. These two changes led to a weight loss of 11 pounds over 16 weeks.

Know when to stop eating: The Appetite Pendulum™

Using my Appetite Pendulum™ is the key to appetite retraining. With practice, you will learn to stop eating a meal when you get to +3 (just full).

The plus numbers on the Appetite Pendulum™ are the ones you tune in to *as you are eating*.

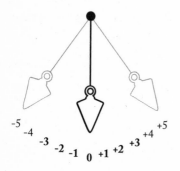

+5 uncomfortably full
+4 very full
+3 just full
+2 nearly full
+1 not sure, probably not hungry
** 0 neutral**
-1 not sure, probably a bit hungry
-2 slightly hungry
-3 definitely hungry
-4 very hungry
-5 extremely hungry

»   +1 feels less like fullness and more like no longer feeling hungry – you've taken the edge off your hunger.

»   + 2 is when you are starting to feel slightly satisfied by your food.

»   +3 is a feeling of definite satisfaction, but not what you're probably used to thinking of as 'full', even though you now need to mentally re-label this state as 'just full'.

»   + 4 tends to feel slightly uncomfortable in your belly while you are eating, but it can be easily overlooked and only registered after a short while – 10–20 minutes later you think 'I didn't need that pudding/second helping.'

» +5 is a feeling of being stuffed, where you are having to think about undoing your trousers. The immediate feeling from your stomach is uncomfortable, but the unpleasant feelings of nausea or of feeling drugged only hit you later. Once you are using Appetite Retraining correctly, you'll never hit +5 because you'll be in tune with your appetite.

The more mindfully you eat, the easier it is to notice what's happening. With each mouthful, you monitor the subtle changing sensations in your stomach. The Japanese principle of eating only until you're 80 per cent full is similar to stopping at +3 on the Appetite Pendulum™. According to the Japanese proverb: 'Eight parts of a full stomach sustain the man; the other two sustain the doctor.'

If you haven't been taking much notice of fullness sensations, this will take a bit of practice. Eating slowly will help you to keep tuned in to your fullness signals. Don't expect to get this right immediately if you've been out of practice for years. If you think you're at +3 but you're not sure, you might want to put your knife and fork down and wait a minute then continue for a few more mouthfuls if you're not quite full. If you overshoot and realize you're at +4 before you've stopped eating, use the opportunity to learn what was too much. Notice the size of what you just ate, and make a mental note that this amount was a bit too much. This can help you adjust better to stopping at +3 at your next meal.

If you've been overeating at mealtimes for years, and doubt whether you can gauge your hunger/fullness level, you can follow everything in the next section, but instead of monitoring your Appetite Pendulum™ number in point 7 serve a different-sized portion. I suggest reducing the size of your meal by a quarter at the start, and for point 7 label how your stomach feels at the end of that meal – '+3 (just full)'.

Whether you're going to monitor your stomach sensations as you eat or reduce the size of your meal by a quarter before you start, you'll be doing this day-in, day-out, so you'll gradually get used to it. It's a process of learning what works – if the new amount is too much or too little, leaving you too hungry or too full, keep playing with the amount until you get it right. Now you know what point you're aiming to stop eating, let's look at how to put this into practice.

Save money
By learning to eat just as much as your body needs, you will eat less so you will spend less.

How to reduce your meal size

1. Work out what to do after you stop eating

When a mouse eats that is all it is doing. Its movement involves putting food into its mouth repeatedly. Once it has had enough, the behaviour switches to grooming and now it just wipes its nose with its paws for a while. The mouse is a valuable role model for us. When you stop eating, you will need to switch to doing something else. Plan what you are going to do as soon as you finish eating and make sure that it is something you can just go and do. It is preferable to do something that occupies your mind and your hands at the same time, such as housework or a hobby. Be aware that watching TV is a very passive activity and it will be easy for your mind to wander to food, particularly because there is so much shown and advertised on TV. It is fine to watch TV as long as you're doing something else at the same time, such as doing a puzzle or a household task. Note that the activity needs to take you away from eating. For example, if you would normally start the washing-up after eating but that means you are in the kitchen being tempted by food, it may be important to leave it until later and do something else in the meantime.

This concrete planning really pays dividends. It's used in elite sport psychology. Soccer player Ronaldinho doesn't just improve his goal-scoring by getting out there on the pitch and practising shots at goal from every conceivable angle. Though of course he does do that. He super-charges this real-life practice by mentally rehearsing the goal-scoring sequence. Here it is in his own words, from an interview with the journalist John Carlin for the *The New York Times*:

'When I train, one of the things I concentrate on is creating a mental picture of how best to deliver the ball to a teammate, preferably leaving him alone in front of the rival goalkeeper. So what I do, always before a game – always, every night and every day – is try and think up things, imagine plays, which no one else will have thought of, and to do so always bearing in mind the particular strength of each teammate to whom I am passing the ball. When I construct those plays in my mind I take into account whether one teammate likes to receive the ball at his feet or ahead of him, if he's good with his head and how he prefers to head the ball, if he's stronger on his right or his left foot. That's my job. That is what I do. I imagine the game.'

This is your Ronaldinho moment. You need to get your plan clear in your mind, and mentally practise it in advance by visualizing what you'll do once you've finished your meal.

Lewis tended to graze on food while he was clearing up after dinner, as he still felt 'peckish'. Using the Appetite Pendulum™ he realized that as he was +3 by the end of dinner, so feeling 'peckish' had more to do with feeling restless than hungry. He changed his routine by going into another room to play his keyboard straight after dinner, and then tidied the kitchen later. By then he found he

wasn't tempted by leftover food so much and could clear up without
grazing. Playing on his keyboard helped discharge the restlessness.

---

2. Remember what you ate for your last meal

Research shows that you tend to eat less for your evening
meal when you first think about what you had for lunch. So
try pausing to think about what you had for your last meal.

3. Use a smaller plate

How full you feel after eating is influenced by how much you
think you're eating, not just the amount you actually had. Our
perception of the quantity of food on our plate is altered by
what proportion of the plate is covered in food. This 'Delboeuf
Illusion' means that eating the same quantity of food off a
smaller plate feels like more than if that amount is eaten off a
larger plate.

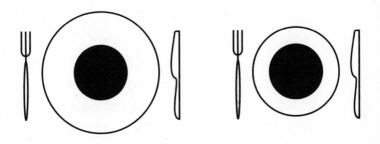

4. Swap your cutlery

You'll be more likely to eat more slowly and therefore eat less if you use just a fork, or use chopsticks instead of the usual knife and fork. Or you could try getting a cutlery set with smaller spoon and fork sizes to help you take smaller mouthfuls.

5. Eat mindfully and maximize pleasure

By paying full attention to what you are eating – eating mindfully – you will notice your changing level of fullness. So sit down to eat rather than standing up or eating on the go and treat the food as important rather than as an afterthought. Eating mindfully means putting your mental focus on the food rather than eating at the same time as doing something else. So turn off the TV and just pay attention. Focus on this mouthful, not the next one. Notice the sight and smell of the food, and as you put the food into your mouth, notice all the textures and flavours. Remember that when you eat food, you get the calories whatever, but you only get all the pleasure that's in that food if you focus on it and eat it mindfully. It is easier to stop eating when your appetite is satisfied. If you really enjoy what you are eating, you get more satisfaction from the same amount of food.

'We miss out on a lot of pleasure when we barely notice the food in our mouth now because we're excitedly looking forward to the next mouthful.'

6. Chew your food well

As you continue chewing, you're likely to notice other flavours coming through. At the start of the 20th century, Horace Fletcher created a craze for chewing food, which had the celebrities of the day hooked on 'Fletcherism' for its impressive health and weight-reducing results. Horace Fletcher became a celebrity of his time, advising American Presidents, British Prime Ministers and some of the big movers and shakers of his age including J. H. Kellogg of the famous cereal company. Even King Edward VII reportedly took up Fletcherizing.

Fletcher argued that we should:

» Chew food until it tastes of nothing, however long that takes.

» Swallow only liquid whilst chewing your food – do not swallow anything solid.

» Whatever solid residue is left in your mouth when there is no taste left should be spat out, never swallowed.

Nowadays that last instruction would get short shrift from dieticians because that's where we get some of the fibre. Although Fletcherism disappeared from view, it may be useful to you in that the more you chew, the slower you eat, and that may give you time to register some of the slower hormonal fullness signals. In fact, recent studies have found that prolonged chewing reduces feelings of hunger and leads to reduced food intake in some people (either in the meal being chewed, or at a later meal). These studies suggest that increasing the number of chews per mouthful of food increases the gut hormones that are involved in registering fullness. Don't worry if you don't want to keep chewing as long as Horace Fletcher did (reportedly upwards of 32 chews per mouthful!); just experiment with chewing longer as a way of helping you to eat less.

7. Monitor your Appetite Pendulum™ number

While you're eating your meal, keep an eye on your Appetite Pendulum™ number (see page 90). Notice the sensations in your stomach changing from hunger to fullness and when you notice that you are just full (+3), STOP EATING and leave the rest. You won't feel physically hungry now, nor will you feel too full. It will probably feel odd to stop eating at this point, especially if you don't like wasting food (see below), but that's okay. It may help to think at this point, 'How will I feel half an hour from now? Will I regret not finishing this food or feel pleased that I stopped?'

8. Notice what you've eaten

When you get to +3, notice the size of what you've eaten to train your eye. This may well come as a shock at first if it's a lot less than you usually eat, and may make you feel uneasy or anxious. If you are +3 on the scale, any discomfort you feel is not physical hunger; it is an emotional reaction to eating less. Dealing with the emotional reactions that eating less produces in you is a crucial part of changing your eating patterns to allow weight loss. There's a section on dealing with anxiety in Chapter 8. In time these feelings will happen less and the new meal size will become your normal meal size.

Noticing the size of your meal is what helps to train your eye to judge the amount your body needs to get to +3 on the Appetite Pendulum™. As you learn this, you can cook/serve/order the right amount of food to start with, so you truly stop wasting food.

9. Move away from the food

Go and do your pre-planned activity (see page 93). You are likely to find that after about 30 minutes, other fullness-related signals have now registered in your brain and the urge to eat more will have lessened. If not, continue with keeping your mind and hands occupied.

10. If it's difficult, use the two-hand interweave

If you're finding it difficult to get away from the food and turn your attention to the activity you planned, the two-hand interweave may help you to resolve this moment of inner conflict. Put 'stop eating now' into one hand, and 'go back for more' in the other and alternately open and close your hands and notice what happens. For more detail on this technique, see page 178.

11. Remember that your next meal will taste fabulous if you stop now

When you stop eating, remind yourself that stopping now means that you'll be able to get hungry by your next meal, so that your taste buds will be sensitized again and the next meal will taste fantastic! If you overeat now and aren't hungry by the next meal, your taste buds won't be sensitive and you'll lose out on the pleasure you could have from that meal. The fear of missing out (FOMO) on the pleasure of this meal is balanced by the greater pleasure of the next. See page 107 for more on this. Also, eating more now would mean eating with desensitized taste buds, so any more of this meal won't taste as good.

12. Menthol mouthwash

Recent studies show that if you wash your mouth out with menthol mouthwash after you've eaten you are less likely to eat again soon. You can use this to your advantage by including it as part of your after-meal routine.

Sarah's overall diet was very healthy, but she wanted to lose some of the weight she'd gained in recent years. She realized that her evening meal had got larger since her husband died and she sometimes felt lonely in the evenings. She didn't want to go on a depriving and miserable diet (wisely), as she'd tried that before with short-term success that was impossible to sustain.

Sarah loved the simplicity and clarity of the Appetite Pendulum™, and particularly the fact that she could eat whatever she liked. She realized that her evening meals had grown in size because she loved the food, and was unsure about reducing the size because she might feel she was depriving herself. To her pleasant surprise, when she used the Appetite Pendulum™ to gauge when to stop eating, she was able to stop at +3 the first time she tried it, and then on several other days the following week. Very quickly she noticed how good she felt about feeling in control of her eating.

By eating mindfully Sarah found that she wasn't feeling deprived as she was getting so much pleasure from what she was eating. This success with her evening meals gave her the confidence to change the timing and size of her lunches, and she lost 6.5kg (14lb) over two months, just from stopping eating her fabulous lunches and dinners when she was just full.

How to enjoy eating desserts

Note: If you are diabetic or pre-diabetic, you should use this section in discussion with your diabetic nurse or doctor.

This section may take some swallowing because it is likely to be at odds with everything you have ever heard about weight loss. With Appetite Retraining, you can include your favourite desserts and still lose weight. You do this by using the Appetite Pendulum™, developing a sharper awareness of when you really have an appetite for something sweet, and by thinking and planning dessert- and sweet-eating. Here are three alternative ways of enjoying desserts:

1. Adjust the size of your main course

Adjust the size of your main course so that you stop eating at +2 on the Appetite Pendulum™ and then eat just enough dessert to take you to +3. This may be difficult to do because both courses would then be very small indeed. If you can deal with this and still stop at +3, all well and good.

2. Eat one meal over two mealtimes

The second way to eat in tune with your body but still have your favourite dessert occasionally is to have only the main course at this meal and only the dessert at the next meal (several hours later when you are -3 on the Appetite Pendulum™). This can be useful for celebratory meals at home where the dessert will still be available several hours later.

If you're eating out and are faced with a large two-course lunch, because of the way your internal clock works (see Chapter 2) you are still likely to want to eat again a few hours later even if you're nowhere near -3 on the Appetite Pendulum™. In this case, the wasted food is whatever you eat in the evening. Spreading the one large lunch over two meals will mean that the -3 to +3 range on the Appetite Pendulum™ can be kept to and excess eating avoided. To do this, ask for a takeaway box for your dessert, or take along your own takeaway box.

3. Have a dessert-only meal

The other possibility is to only eat dessert at this meal. The idea of the dessert-only meal may horrify you, but think about it for a moment. If you really want to eat a dessert but instead you have a savoury meal, the craving for the sweet food may still be there. Many people eat substantial amounts of savoury food in order to feel 'allowed' to have the dessert. In this case the wasted calories are in the savoury food eaten to 'earn' the dessert. Something I find fascinating about helping people to retrain their appetite is that when they really, really let themselves have the cake or whatever it is, they lose the obsession with it. They no longer hanker for it and it becomes something they occasionally fancy.

For any of these options, where you end up with a dessert-only meal, it's crucial to keep aware of your hunger and fullness levels, so that you stop eating the dessert at +3. Given the portion sizes of shop-bought and restaurant portions, this is likely to be half a cake or half the dessert rather than the full portion. So, go prepared with your takeaway box so that you can have the other half another day.

Once you get more practised at gauging whether you really want dessert (see Chapter 9), there are likely to be times when you realize you just want something, not really dessert – just something to end the meal. In this case having a hot drink is a good option. It could be your favourite tea, it could even be hot chocolate. But equally you might find that you just fancy hot water.

Appetite Retraining does *not* advocate eating an unbalanced diet or eating lots of sweet foods. The dessert-only meal will only be a very occasional event. If it is not, you may have developed sugar cravings (see page 198).

The strength of incorporating desserts as part of Appetite Retraining is that when you have reached your goal weight, eating dessert has become established as part of your new eating patterns, in tune with your hunger and appetite and does not need to be re-introduced after a period of abstinence.

Increased confidence
Each time you stop eating at +3, notice what that tells you about yourself. You may not believe it at first, but when you repeatedly succeed at stopping eating at this point of being

just full, your brain will form a new belief that you are capable of being in control around eating. You'll notice a shift in how you see yourself, not only in the mirror, but in terms of self-confidence and self-control.

Wasting food

When you stop eating at +3 there may still be food on your plate. Your next task is to store the leftover meal or throw it in the bin. If you are confident that when it is back in the fridge or larder you can forget about it until your next mealtime, it is fine to put it back. If you suspect that you will be tempted to go and finish it off before you are next hungry, then you will lose weight more quickly if you put it in the bin.

Just about everyone I have worked with using Appetite Retraining has initially gasped in horror at the suggestion of throwing food away. What I explain is this:

» Your body digests the food you eat at each meal and uses the energy produced to get you through the next few hours. If there is any extra energy left by the time of your next meal, it converts it into fat. So all the extra (unnecessary) food you ate at your last meal becomes fat.

» Food is certainly no less wasted if it goes through your body and is converted into fat than if it goes straight into the bin. Putting it in the bin does not make you fat and doesn't have adverse side-effects on your health.

» If you keep eating up food you don't need, you keep wasting it. And you gain extra weight.

You won't need to throw much food in the bin before you get the hang of how much your body needs at a particular mealtime to get you to +3. Thus, the net result of Appetite Retraining is that you will waste *less* food than you have in the past. In particular, you will waste less food by putting it through your body to be stored as extra fat.

'When you repeatedly succeed at stopping eating at this point of being just full, your brain will form a new belief that you are capable of being in control around eating.'

How to deal with the Fear of Missing Out (FOMO)

One of the reasons for eating meals that are much bigger than we need is that we are eating for pleasure, or at least trying to. Eating for pleasure is a good thing and we are biologically programmed to find food pleasurable. When you are enjoying a meal or snack, you tend to want to keep eating more of it. This means that when you get to +3 on the Appetite Pendulum™, you will have to give up some pleasure by stopping eating.

However, as you eat any particular dish, your taste buds become gradually less sensitive to that food. This is one of the ways our appetite is regulated. When you eat beyond +3 on the Appetite Pendulum™, the law of diminishing returns kicks in: you will get less pleasure from each successive bite as your taste sensitivity decreases. Most of the pleasure is in the first half of the meal.

Here, it helps to remember that when you stop at +3 you are helping your next meal to taste delicious because you will be hungry by your next mealtime. As Mireille Guiliano in *French Women Don't Get Fat* says:

'One thing French women know is that the pleasure of most foods is in the first few bites; we rarely have seconds.'

So, the pleasure you give up by stopping at +3, you gain back in effect at the next meal because that meal will be more enjoyable if you are hungry when you start eating. Overall with Appetite Retraining you are likely to get more pleasure from food rather than less because you will be eating foods you love, when your taste buds are at their most sensitive.

'Because your taste bud sensitivity reduces bite by bite, the second half of a meal is less tasty than the first. By eating less at this meal, you allow your body to get hungry by the next, so that meal will taste fabulous. What you miss out at this meal in pleasure, you gain at the next.'

How to stop binge eating

Bingeing refers to eating a large amount of food in a way that feels out of control. It tends to happen to people who engage in very restrictive diets, because restricting what and how much you eat, puts your body under increasingly strong physiological pressure to eat. It is also more common in people who place a high value on weight and shape and in people who are prone to emotional eating.

Binges tend to be triggered by:
» Breaking a dietary rule
» Alcohol or drugs
» An external event
» A negative mood state

To reduce bingeing, make sure that you don't wait to eat until you are excessively hungry. Space your meals and choose what to eat so that you get to -3 (definitely hungry) by the next meal. Don't wait to eat until you are -4 or -5 on the Appetite Pendulum™, because that would make binge eating more likely to happen. For more on how to deal with emotional eating, see Chapter 8.

If you find that your binge eating nevertheless continues, I recommend reading *Overcoming Binge Eating* by Dr Christopher Fairburn, an international authority on binge eating. Dr Fairburn's book is a guided self-help programme using up-to-date cognitive behavioural techniques, which helps you to overcome binge eating step by step. If your binge eating is out of control, you may be suffering from Binge-Eating Disorder. The diagnostic criteria for the condition are given on page 281. This recognized mental health condition is likely to need professional intervention and you should in the first instance talk to your GP about how to get help.

Bulimia Nervosa

Binge-Eating Disorder is different from Bulimia Nervosa as it does not involve purging. If you are struggling with bingeing and purging, you may be suffering from Bulimia Nervosa and again this is something which may require professional help and you should discuss this with your GP. If you are bingeing and purging, the purging is likely to be a reaction to the bingeing, so anything that helps reduce the binges is likely also to help reduce the urge to purge.

'We're bombarded with encouragement to eat more than we need. Taking back control of how much we eat is one of the best things we can do not just for our weight, but for our overall health too.'

Learning how to stop eating when you're just full is a cornerstone of Appetite Retraining, because eating beyond that point is, for many of us, exactly what keeps us heavier than we want to be. Whether that's because your meal sizes are too big or you can't resist desserts or you tend to binge eat, discovering how to adjust the amount you eat is key to losing weight and keeping it off.

Don't expect overnight success if you've been in the habit of overeating for a long time. Take one step at a time, using any of the techniques I've given on pages 93 to 100. Bring your best benefit to mind every time you feel your motivation flagging. If stopping eating at 'just full' is making you feel anxious, find an anxiety reduction technique from those on pages 211 to 215 that works for you.

Give yourself credit each time you manage to stop eating at +3 and over a few weeks you will discover that you can learn to eat differently and feel more in control around food and eating.

As you stop eating when you're just full, your meals will be the size your body needs to keep you going for a few hours while you get on with your day. Next we're going to look at how to establish an eating routine for those meals that fits in to your lifestyle, with snacks to tide you over where needed.

CHAPTER 5

—

Establish a New Routine

There are several reasons for getting in to some sort of routine with your eating. First, because of the way your stomach and gut work. In Chapter 2 we learned that the design of the human gut is suited to eating meals spaced at intervals – it's not suited to continual grazing or occasional massive meals. Second, because of the way our internal body clock works. Third, because of evidence that people who keep weight off tend to have a routine for eating.

Professor Jane Wardle's research team, at University College London, found that having a regular eating routine is one of the characteristics of people who successfully keep weight off once they have lost it, which is another reason for getting your eating routine sorted out now. Anything that helps you stay at your new weight, after the effort of getting there, is to be seized on! Having an erratic eating routine isn't a problem for some people. If you were someone who could eat at various times, on the go, and your health was good and your weight comfortable, there wouldn't be an issue. But if you are overeating and you don't have a routine for eating, it will help. Finally, because skipping a meal to try to save calories tends to backfire. If you skip breakfast, for instance, so you'll have more 'calorie-allowance' left for the evening, you're trying to manage your weight by your head, not your gut. And ignoring your gut is what got you where you are today! If you miss a meal because of circumstances, or because you're totally immersed in something, don't worry but do try to re-establish your eating routine afterwards.

What sort of routine do you need?

There is no one eating routine that suits everyone, so you can work out what times of meals and snacks suit *your* lifestyle. Most people have three meals a day, though some prefer to have two, while others prefer to eat more often. The emphasis with Appetite Retraining is on making changes to your eating habits that are easy for you personally to stick to. Whatever routine you develop for yourself, it needs to fit around your lifestyle so that it's easy to keep to. Aim to leave a few hours between meals. As you'll see, if your lifestyle means that there is sometimes too long a gap between two meals that might risk taking you beyond -3 on the Appetite Pendulum™, then you can timetable in a snack to tide you over.

Your routine doesn't have to be the same every day. Many people have a different routine on working days than they do on non-working days so you may have to adapt your pattern as necessary.

'Having regular meals that are the right size to give you the energy you need for a few hours means you'll enjoy every meal.'

What will your new eating routine be?

Remember that as a human being you have a digestive system that has evolved to eat a quantity of food to provide energy for the next few hours' activity. You are not a cow or sheep that needs to graze for large parts of its waking life. Nor are you a snake that can eat once every few days on an enormous and hard-to-digest prey.

With Appetite Retraining your new mealtime routines will reflect your body's basic biology of eating so that you eat enough to keep you going for a few hours at a time. Eating times will fit into your real-life routine, including family mealtimes, business lunches, and times when you particularly eat for pleasure.

Being able to leave gaps between meals during which you become definitely hungry by the start of your next meal allows:

1. Weight loss
2. Increased taste bud sensitivity so that your next meal tastes fantastic!
3. Some of the health benefits that come from fasting, such as your gut starting to clean itself (see Chapter 2).

How to adjust your eating routine

First of all, using the table below, jot down the times you eat meals and have snacks. You may not eat three meals and three snacks a day – just fill in what you do currently.

Existing routine

	Mon	Tues	Wed	Thurs	Fri	Sat	Sun
Breakfast							
Morning snack							
Lunch							
Afternoon snack							
Dinner							
Evening snack							

Now look at your chart.

» What do you notice?

» How often do you miss breakfast?

» Do you skip lunch?

Dominic had identified his first Unhelpful Eating Habit: his evening meal was too large. He was in a pattern of buying take-away food on the way home and then eating a meal with his family when he got in. He wanted to be able to eat less in the evenings in order to lose weight. He worked as a development manager for a growing chain of retail shops, which involved preparing new shops for opening and training up new staff teams to work in them. The work was full-on, and he realized that on working days he often didn't have time to think about food. When we looked at this in more detail, Dominic was astonished to realize that from when he finished the family meal at 8pm until buying his takeaway at 6.30pm the next evening, he was eating virtually nothing. He was bewildered that he hadn't realized this before! It made complete sense to him then why he ate so much in the evenings as he was ravenously hungry by then.

On the next page is another table for you to sketch out rough times for meals (and snacks if needed), which would give you a more regular routine than the one you filled in above. As I said earlier, you may need different routines for different types of days, but it doesn't matter as long as you're spacing out your meals, but not going too long without food.

The chart doesn't have to be perfect – it's a working document – and you'll need to use trial and error to discover the sizes and types of meals that will fit your eating routine. If a highlight of your day is an evening treat, include that in your new routine. Cutting out a much-looked-forward-to indulgence in the evening or trying to replace it with something that doesn't feel indulgent at all could easily feel like deprivation and set you up to fail. You may need to change the size and alter the timing of the treat in order to enjoy it and lose weight, or change the timing or size of your evening meal.

New routine

	Mon	Tues	Wed	Thurs	Fri	Sat	Sun
Breakfast							
Morning snack							
Lunch							
Afternoon snack							
Dinner							
Evening snack							

Zoe was a student living with her mother. She had suffered for a number of years with anorexia nervosa and wanted to lose weight without triggering a recurrence of the eating disorder. She was gaining weight and starting to feel out of control around eating again. It really mattered to her to find something that would work for her. When she looked at her routine, she realized that by waiting to eat with her mother at about 8pm, she'd got into the habit of eating snacks to keep her going. This meant that by dinnertime she wasn't that hungry, but ate the meal anyway. Zoe decided to approach her mother about eating dinner much earlier, at 6pm, which her mother agreed they could do. On evenings when Zoe was at home, she had a small dessert with her mother at about 9pm, which seemed to suit them both. This change of timing of her evening meal meant that Zoe was no longer snacking in the run-up to dinner, and regaining control of her eating was the first in a series of steps which allowed her to lose 14kg (31lb) and keep it off, without triggering a recurrence of her eating disorder. In fact, she said that she now felt more relaxed around food.

Using your new routine

You're aiming to have regular meals spaced a few hours apart. The size of each meal and what sort of food you eat influences how long it will take for your body to digest it and feel hungry again. Protein and fats keep us fuller for longer, so if you've got a longer gap between, say breakfast and lunch, try having these foods for breakfast, such as scrambled eggs or avocado on toast. Vegetables and fruit tend to be digested more quickly leaving you feeling hungry sooner, so they are ideal for a snack when it's only an hour or two until your next meal.

Before the overweight epidemic, this is how people tended to eat – they did not have as many snacks as we do now. So, try eating meals at these regular times for a few days and see what happens. Be prepared that you may encounter feelings of hunger and/or anxiety at times.

Dealing with hunger

If you start to feel hungry between meals, that's great. As your hunger increases, notice it and remind yourself that this feeling of hunger is a signal that your body is shifting from digesting its last meal to burning up some stored fat. This is what you want, so this mild hunger is to be embraced rather than avoided or dreaded. Also, whenever you feel hungry between meals, this is a reminder to look forward with pleasure to your next meal knowing that it will taste fabulous because your taste buds will be at their most sensitive.

If you get to -3 (definitely hungry) on the Appetite Pendulum™ more than an hour before your next meal, have a snack. Keep the snack small (enough to get you to +2) so that you allow yourself to get to -3 again by the time of the next meal. You will learn after doing this a few times what size of snack takes the edge off your hunger but allows you to get to -3 by the next meal. A good snack for these purposes is a piece of fresh fruit, although a banana may keep you going for longer so if this is your favourite fruit it may be best to eat only half of it. If you're definitely hungry and it's a couple of hours or more before your next meal, find a snack that will keep you going for longer, such as a handful of nuts or a piece of cheese with apple.

This is new, so don't expect yourself to get it right all the time. Keep experimenting and you will find out what works.

Dealing with anxiety

Like many people, you may feel anxious or uncomfortable when you are hungry, or even when you are not hungry, and eat to try to relieve it. With Appetite Retraining you can learn to deal with anxiety directly and not by using food. To discover your best anxiety-reduction technique, choose the one that works best for you in the section 'How to Deal with Anxiety' in Chapter 8 (see pages 211–215). If you are tempted to eat between meals from now on, but are not hungry, use your chosen anxiety-reduction technique *and* distract yourself with something else.

The importance of keeping occupied

For many people, overeating is a response to under-activity and boredom. If this applies to you, you need to make sure you have some activities to engage in between meals, such as hobbies, interests, chores, social contact, admin tasks and work. If you don't already have things to do when you are not eating, have one or more (preferably a few) things you have ready to do to distract you from thoughts of eating.

You may need different distractions at times of day. For example, when you're tired you'll need some low-energy distractions such as doing a puzzle, surfing the internet, doing a relaxing craft activity, reading or watching TV. When you're feeling more energetic, you could garden, exercise, do chores or learn a new language for distraction.

Skimping on meals

If the meal you eat is too small, it can act as an appetizer and stimulate, rather than satisfy, your desire to eat. This is why meals stop at 'just full' (+3 on the Appetite Pendulum™). Also, if you eat a meal that takes you to less than +3, you will be hungry again sooner and this is likely to interfere with your overall routine. For these reasons, use +3 on the Appetite Pendulum™ as the measure of when you have eaten enough. The Appetite Pendulum™ is a subjective scale. This is deliberate. You need to gauge what is happening in your body. If you are getting too hungry too soon after a meal, you need to recalibrate things so that you eat a bit more and call the feeling you get then, 'just full' (+3). If you aren't losing weight, then you need to recalibrate things so that you eat smaller meals and call the feeling you get then 'just full' (+3).

Skipping breakfast or other meals

With Appetite Retraining, skipping breakfast is not helpful if you're doing it to try and 'save' calories for later. Breakfast helps to re-set your internal body clock and it provides the fuel for the morning. Skipping breakfast can make weight loss harder because your energy levels may dip and leave you less able to use willpower later in the day. Skipping lunch is likely to leave you with depleted fuel for the afternoon and may lead to your eating becoming more erratic later on.

The other consequence of skipping breakfast or lunch is that you can become too hungry (-4 or -5 on the Appetite Pendulum™) by the next mealtime. Then there is a tendency to overeat at the next meal, which in turn upsets the whole gentle regulation of appetite and eating. If you have skipped meals in the past, resolve to re-introduce regular meals so that you can eat in the way your body is designed for.

Many people tell me that they don't eat breakfast because they're not hungry first thing. This is often because they are eating too much in the evenings. Altering your evening eating pattern can allow you to get hungry by breakfast, which will then taste fabulous. If it suits you, and you prefer not to have breakfast in the early morning your first meal of the day will then be later on, and provided that you adjust meal sizes and content so that you are definitely hungry by each meal and just full at the end of each meal (with snacks to tide you over if needed), you'll be fine.

Anna arrived home from work at 5.30pm and snacked on anything to hand whilst she and her husband cooked together and talked about their day. This, and then eating together, were her favourite times of day and she did not want to spoil this by having to follow a different diet from her husband. Besides, she was tired when she got in and cooking one meal was quite enough.

Using the Appetite Pendulum™ Anna was able to see that by the time she arrived home from work she was usually ravenous (−5). In the hour it took to get dinner ready, she would pick at food without realizing it. It also showed that although she had a healthy lunch at a regular time of 12.30pm, she was definitely hungry (−3) by mid-afternoon. Her lunch wasn't enough to keep her going until her evening meal, but because of wanting to lose weight, Anna felt she shouldn't snack during the afternoon to avoid extra calories. Anna needed to be less hungry by the time she got home, so that she could prepare the meal without picking at food, and then really enjoy dinner with her husband. Anna chose to take to work a small pack of nuts or a piece of cheese with celery or a piece of bread and honey, to eat at about 4pm. This meant she could focus on cooking without picking at food and wait to eat until dinner was ready. This, and using a smaller plate at dinner time, led Anna to lose 4kg (9lb) over two months.

In the next chapter we'll look at the ways in which our subconscious minds can scupper our efforts to keep to a new eating routine and change our unhelpful eating habits.

CHAPTER 6

—

Tackle Your Saboteurs

Not everyone finds themselves sabotaging their progress when they try to lose weight, but it's very common, particularly among people who've tried to lose weight and failed in the past. If this has happened to you, this chapter will be important to work through.

As I described in Chapter 1, mental blocks are those puzzling and annoying hurdles to weight loss that tend to kick in after the initial honeymoon period of any diet. Working as a Clinical Psychologist, I'm used to people coming up against hurdles when they try to make changes in their lives. Inner resistance to change is natural and normal. As I developed Appetite Retraining, I soon saw self-sabotage in action and I worked on trying to make sense of it for clients. I started to collect all the reasons people were giving me for why diets hadn't worked for them in the past, and why they sometimes had difficulty changing even just one eating habit at a time when they were working with me.

The reasons they gave boiled down to 29 statements, and I eventually categorized these hurdles into four types. We'll look at each of these types in this chapter and I'll give you concrete tips for how to overcome them.

> **'Overcoming each weight-loss hurdle doesn't only allow our body to shed pounds; it allows us to discover strengths and abilities we didn't know we had.'**

Why can't you succeed in losing weight?

The four types of saboteurs can crop up in relation to eating even if you are super-successful in other areas of your life. So if you're usually able to achieve goals you set yourself and succeed with flying colours, why can't you stick to your eating plan? Trouble changing your eating habits isn't to do with ability or intelligence. Oprah Winfrey is one of the most successful people on TV and she openly talks about her struggles with losing weight and gaining it again. You, me, Oprah – we all encounter hurdles when we try and change something as fundamental as how we eat. Hurdles put there by the subconscious part of our mind. Each of us can overcome our hurdles when we understand what they are and what specifically we need to do to get over them.

It's often because losing weight is more complicated psychologically speaking than you may think, and that complexity is to do with the unconscious part of our mind. That's what saboteurs are – the psychological processes influencing how we eat that aren't conscious. But being able to anticipate what natural blocks or saboteurs are likely to crop up means that you can bring them into your conscious mind and deal with them directly. Forewarned is fore-armed.

The first step is to understand what is getting in your way. The second is to learn how to overcome it.

Understand your own self-sabotage

To understand your own hurdles to losing weight and being able to keep it off easily, take a look at the following Saboteurs statements and tick all those that apply to you.

The four sections refer to the four different types of saboteur that I identified as I developed Appetite Retraining. The more items you ticked in each section, the more of an issue that type of saboteur is likely to be for you. I'll explain what each of the saboteur types is, and then how you can deal with any that apply to you, so that you don't find yourself undoing the progress you make.

All the statements on the next 29 pages are examples of why weight loss failed previously for clients I've worked with. Decide which statements apply to you and tick the box on those pages. Then on page 163, you'll summarize which saboteur statements apply to you.

A

☐

I don't want to put
        my life on hold
while I go on a diet.

☐

Part of me wants
to lose weight;
another part just
can't be bothered
and just wants to
enjoy food.

A

☐

Being overweight gives
me something to focus
my worrying on.
If I'm slim,
I'll have to tackle the
more difficult problems
in my life.

☐

If I successfully
lose weight, I'll have
to cope with
being more sexually
attractive/cope with
intimacy.

A

☐

Eating what I want
when I want
is the only thing I can
control in my life.

☐

Others will envy me if
    I successfully lose weight
and I won't be able
    to cope
       with that.

A

☐

I have too much else
going on in my life
right now to focus on
weight loss.

☐

I feel guilty
    when I eat
nice food.

B

☐

Because I'm already
overweight,
I don't deserve
to eat
nice food.

☐

I've been overweight
so long that I won't feel
like me if
I successfully
lose weight.

B

☐

I don't
deserve to be slim, happy
or successful.

☐

I'm so overweight,
I will never
be able to lose weight.

☐

I always fail at diets,
so I'll fail
at this.
No diet can help me.

☐

I have no
willpower/I am a weak
person.

C

☐

I'm OK in the week
when I'm busy,
but then my eating
goes to pot at weekends.

☐

Once I start
eating,
I can't stop.

c

☐

I'm good in the
mornings, but
hopeless in
the evenings,
when I can't resist eating.

☐

I can't
resist cravings for
particular
foods.

C

☐

I can control my eating until I see some tempting food and then I don't care whether I'm overweight and I just eat it.

C

☐

I can't resist eating
a snack when
I have a drink
(of tea, coffee, alcohol etc).

C

☐

I can't get motivated
to make the effort
to lose weight.

☐

I haven't got the
self-discipline
to eat the right
foods.

D

☐

My partner/mother/friend
cooks for me.
If I don't
eat the meals,
I'll be offending them.

☐

My partner
prefers me this weight
so doesn't want me
to lose weight.

D

☐

I feel I have to stay
overweight to fit
in to my family or
social circle and remain
loyal to them and to my
place in that group.

☐

When I'm with X
    even if I'm not hungry
s/he wants me
    to eat with her/him and
      I feel bad if I refuse.

D

☐

Other people
put pressure on me
to eat more.

☐

In social situations
other people push more
food on to
me than I want.
They make me feel like a
party-pooper
if I don't join in.

D

☐

There's
   someone important
        to me in my life
   who wants me to
        lose weight

Reading your results

Check and note down how many statements you chose from the pages marked:

A ....

B ....

C ....

D ....

Now turn to the pages that are most relevant to you for specific advice on addressing your potential hurdles head-on. The more items you've checked for each saboteur type, the more relevant that saboteur is likely to be for you.

Section A is about Ambivalence

Ambivalence is about holding two conflicting but true thoughts or feelings at the same time, such as wanting to lose weight but at the same time not really being that bothered. It produces wavering commitment to achieving your goal. Ambivalence about losing weight can produce fluctuating motivation, so that sometimes you are determined to succeed and other times it doesn't seem to matter. If this applies to you, read pages 165–168.

Section B is about Self-Belief

As Henry Ford said, 'Whether you believe you can do something or believe you can't, you're probably right.' What we believe about ourselves often becomes a self-fulfilling prophecy, so if you seriously doubt your ability to lose weight, it's more likely that you'll fail. The self-belief items in Section B include self-esteem, self-image and self-efficacy, which are different aspects of believing in your ability to achieve a goal. If this applies to you, read pages 169–175.

Section C is about Willpower

Lacking willpower means not having mental energy when you need it, which leads to a lack of focus at those moments. For example, you might cave in to having seconds when you were crystal-clear about portion sizes earlier. If this applies to you, read pages 176–179.

Section D is about Pressure from other people around eating

If other people get involved, losing weight isn't just your own private battle. Even if they're trying to help, pressure from people you care about can make things more difficult. If this applies to you, read pages 180–182.

How to overcome your ambivalence

If you genuinely want to lose weight and genuinely don't, for whatever reason, at some point this conflict will surface. Usually as I've said, it comes to light after you start to diet, a few weeks in (or days if the diet is too extreme). It starts to feel like too much and you fall back off the wagon, and back to how you normally eat.

This works the other way around as well. If you are truly ambivalent about weight loss, before long you'll be unhappy with this and will find yourself thinking again about your next diet. Real ambivalence about anything results in dithering or prevarication – a repetitive cycle of half-doing then undoing the same thing. This can of course apply to other areas of your life too.

If you're a serial dieter, this may be exactly what's been happening. In which case this section is really important for you. The simple exercises here will help you get out of your dieting limbo.

1. The bench overlooking the sea

Remember that ambivalence arises from having two conflicting desires simultaneously. You can think of these as different parts of yourself. One part that wants to lose weight and another part that doesn't and just wants to enjoy as much lovely food as possible. This exercise will help you discover what these two parts of you are actually conflicted about and what you can do to reduce the conflict.

First imagine the two parts of you like two separate people sitting on a bench on the seafront together looking out to sea. You can fill in the details of the scene to make it just as you'd like the view to be. As you sit and watch the world go by, take it in turns to talk about dieting and why it hasn't worked before, and how you could make it work in future. The key is for each part to talk just about their point of view and for the other part to listen respectfully. Let each side have their say, in turn and keep going until each side has said all they want to. This way you move away from the battle and towards diplomacy! Whatever you do around food, the two sides need to co-operate. If each one's viewpoint is taken into consideration, it's more likely this can happen.

Then, try getting the two sides to agree on a compromise of just focusing on one eating habit change at a time. It may help you to focus just on reducing the size of your evening meal by a quarter, every day. The food-loving side of you will be happy to eat delicious food and the part that wants to lose weight will be happy with reducing the meal size. Once you get used to doing this and it feels easy, you can plan your next step-change in eating habits. And remember to involve both parts of yourself in the planning. Any time you need to, go back to that imaginary bench on the seafront and listen to what each side of you thinks. When you make progress and give both sides credit for the achievement, you'll be able to feel happier and stronger. And whatever you do, acknowledge the two sides of yourself and the fact that both need to be taken into account.

2. Strengthen and develop your goal daily

Changing how you eat takes effort and focus. You need to be clear about your goal and keep that at the forefront of your mind during the time it takes to lose the weight. Keeping your goal in mind will help you keep going, and will help you get there. Think of when you've revised for an exam. It probably wasn't the enjoyment of revising that kept your nose to the grindstone; it was your desire to get a good grade. If it weren't for wanting the goal, you'd probably give up.

To strengthen your awareness of your goal, spend some time with it. Try to do the Best Benefit visualization technique (see pages 74–6) once every day for two minutes from now until your weight loss is established and you no longer need it. Choose the visualization that relates to your best benefit: looking good, feeling fit and healthy or feeling confident.

Doing this two-minute visualization every day will help you to tune in to the bigger picture and get to know your future slimmer self. This particularly matters if you're anxious about how losing weight and changing shape may affect you and your relationships. The visualization means that you gradually get used to what it's going to be like to succeed, and you can gradually get your head around how this will feel. You'll need to let yourself feel good about making progress. You'll need to handle feelings of pride about how you look or how strong you are. It may sound crazy for me to warn you to prepare for success, but our brains like what's familiar, even if that is negative. So when you prove that you can do something that you didn't believe you could, it can feel weird or even wrong. And then your brain will work to square the circle either by updating your view of yourself, or by reverting to your familiar 'failed dieter' persona. This chapter is all about making sure it's the first of these.

As you spend a couple of minutes each day doing this Best Benefit visualization exercise, you'll be strengthening your connection with your goal. This has two particular benefits: first, it makes it easier to conjure up an image of why you are making the effort to change your eating habits whenever you're tempted to stop. Second, by getting to know your future self, you won't be surprised when you become him or her. It will feel natural and familiar. And your brain will like that.

'You need to be clear about your goal and keep that at the forefront of your mind.'

How to increase your self-belief

It is much easier to achieve a goal if you believe that you can do it. We derive belief in our ability to do something (self-efficacy) from previous successes. We expect failure where we have failed before. This is intelligent learning from experience. If you've failed at dieting before, your self-belief may be low. Some hard facts may help you here.

In the USA, the National Weight Control Registry (NWCR) has 3,000 names. To get on to this register, the person must have lost at least 13.5kg (30lb) and kept it off for over a year. Impressively, the *average* weight loss among the 3,000 listed people is 30kg (66lb) kept off for an average of six years! Over 90 per cent of people on the list had previously tried to lose weight, so these very successful losers were previously 'failed dieters'. This shows that there are successful and unsuccessful weight-loss attempts rather than successful and unsuccessful dieters.

The study also showed that nearly half the people had been overweight before the age of 11 so having longstanding excess weight does not prevent success. Almost half of the 3,000 people had one parent who was overweight and over a quarter had two overweight parents, which shows that even a possible genetic tendency to being overweight in the family does not prevent successful weight loss and maintenance.

There are different types of self-doubt when it comes to believing you will be able to succeed at losing weight permanently. The three most common are:

» 'I don't deserve to lose weight.'
» 'It doesn't feel safe for me to lose weight.'
» 'I won't feel like me if I lose weight.'

We'll take each of these in turn.

I don't deserve to lose weight

This is all about self-esteem. Negative beliefs about yourself develop on the basis of experience, either while you were growing up or more recently during adulthood. There are many different types of experience that can produce low self-esteem, but what people with low self-esteem have in common is that they have come to believe that they themselves are defective or bad, irrespective of whether there is any truth to this.

Unfortunately, once this belief has taken hold, you tend to behave as though it were true and other people then tend to treat you accordingly. Feeling undeserving can become a self-fulfilling prophecy: you think you don't deserve anything good, so you don't claim good things when they are available and may even turn down good things that are offered. Other people can find this puzzling, particularly when they really like and value you. You can take either of two approaches here.

1.   Allow the possibility that your beliefs about not deserving good things could be mistaken. Gently starting to lose weight is a way of finding out what it feels like to make positive changes in your life. Taking things slowly and recognizing how odd and uncomfortable eating nice food and losing weight feels, may help you to start building your self-esteem one step at a time.

2.   If the self-esteem issue feels so significant that it would sabotage any success you have, you could put weight loss on hold just for now and do work on your self-esteem first. See Resources, page 275.

Harriet had a longstanding sense of inferiority compared with other people. She knew logically that she had a good job and nice house and was in a good relationship, but her self-esteem had always been low. She was a very competent person, and when she quickly grasped the principles of Appetite Retraining, she started to make good progress, but this soon faltered. We shifted our attention to her saboteurs, which were mainly lack of self-belief and lack of willpower. It turned out that the two were connected, because feeling inferior to others meant she always put them first. She was convinced that other people were superior to her and therefore deserved more. However tired Harriet was, she would go the extra mile for her employer and work late.

For Harriet, increasing willpower meant enhancing her self-esteem and self-belief first. As we talked, a penny dropped for Harriet for the first time in her life, and with a huge smile she *said, 'Wow! I've just realized that no other f***** has got any more idea about life than I have!' This insight was a turning point that enabled Harriet to have the confidence to see herself on a level with others, which meant that she slowly began to believe that she was as entitled as anyone else to eat lovely things. She stopped eating in secret and began looking after herself better, first of all by leaving work at 5pm rather than working hours of unpaid overtime. In turn this meant that she had the energy (willpower) to make positive changes to her eating patterns.*

It doesn't feel safe to lose weight

If, even subconsciously, we don't think it will be safe to do something, our hard-wired survival mechanisms kick in to keep us from doing it. Safety is the most basic human function of all. Even more than eating or having sex, staying safe always trumps everything else because in evolutionary terms, safety was the same thing as staying alive. Many of the things we experience as threatening in modern life aren't mortal threats, but social threats operate using the same biological systems in our bodies that deal with life-or-death dangers. We may feel absolutely terrified of giving a talk in public even though the worst that can happen is that people think our talk was rubbish. The reason for social threats being so serious is itself an evolutionary thing – being cast out of our social group was a mortal threat during earlier stages of human evolution. But with a public-speaking fear, that's not the case. Subconscious fears about whether it will be okay to lose weight are rather like the public speaking example, and they can produce just as much terror. When it comes to losing weight, there are three areas in particular that can scare people. These are:

Having to deal with other big issues in your life

Being unhappy with your weight can be all-consuming, leaving you with little mental bandwidth to think about what else is going on in your life. At times this may be useful. If you have a major issue that is too painful to think about, either in the present or from the past, obsessing about eating might help keep the more difficult things out of your mind. If this is the case, give yourself permission to decide whether now is a good time to work on losing weight or not. It may be better to acknowledge what's been holding you back and decide to postpone weight loss until you feel equipped to tackle the issues you've been avoiding. Or you may want to go ahead and change how you eat now. Either way, now you have recognized the existence of something so difficult, it may be a good time to seek help from a friend or professional (see Resources, page 275) to work out how to approach dealing with it.

Having to deal with intimacy

Although intimacy is something we may long for, it isn't always straightforward. If part of the reason you overeat is fear that you'll have to cope with physical or emotional intimacy if you slim down, that fear is likely to surface as your weight starts dropping. As with other fears, you can either take the weight loss steps gradually, feeling your way with issues around intimacy as you go, or work on the intimacy issue first and put losing weight on hold until it feels less scary.

Having to deal with other people's envy

Envy is the feeling we get when someone else has something we want but don't have. Envy makes us want to destroy that thing for the other person as it is too painful to see them with it. If a friend envies your ability to lose weight, s/he may do things to prevent you succeeding, such as pushing food on you when you don't want it. Fear of others' envy can prevent us reaching our potential in life. Notice that launching into trying to lose weight while you are afraid of provoking envy means that as you succeed, you will get scared. You may want to recruit help with this, either by confiding in a non-envious friend or relative to help you with these feelings as they emerge or by finding a therapist. If someone can help you with those fearful feelings as you successfully lose weight, you can work out how your relationship with the person who envies you can change. If it can't change, you need to decide whether weight loss is worth the impact on your relationship with them.

'Confirmation Bias is the tendency to unconsciously attend to information that fits what we already believe and discount what doesn't. To change, we have to be open to signs that our existing beliefs about

ourselves may be mistaken. We may be
stronger than we thought.'

I won't feel like me if I lose weight

This is about your self-image. We get used to how we look. When
we start to look different, mental energy is required to adjust to the
new appearance. By 'adjust' I mean come to feel comfortable with.

Imagine that you got rid of all your existing clothes and
went and bought a whole new wardrobe in an entirely new
style. You might like the new style, or not. It might suit you,
or not. Other people may react differently to you in your new
outfits. However positive the new look is, it will feel weird to
begin with. Probably nice-weird.

Losing weight is a bit like this. The more sudden the weight
loss, the more energy it takes to get to feel comfortable again
with how you look. Gradual change is easier to adjust to, but
even then it does take some getting used to. Chapter 10 talks
about adjusting to your new size and weight. You don't need to
do anything more with this at this stage other than note that we
will take adjusting to your new weight into account. There are
people who have lost huge amounts of weight by dieting who
have put it back on because they did not feel themselves at this
new weight.

Go gently with getting used to your body changing and
talk to people you trust about any doubts you have about your
new shape.

How to tackle a lack of willpower

To understand the role of willpower in losing weight, it helps to realize that success results from a series of moments – decision points – rather than a continuous slog. It's those few seconds that crop up when you are about to do the old thing (such as keep eating beyond the point of being just full), but need to do the new thing (stop eating now) instead. At each of these brief decision points, more energy is needed to do the new thing than the old thing, but only briefly. Once you've done that new thing, you just get on with the next thing in your day. So you need to make it as easy as possible to do the new, higher-energy, thing.

Understanding willpower

Willpower isn't what you may think. It's not a personality trait, or a failing. It's more like a type of energy. In their book *Willpower*, Roy Baumeister and John Tierney summarize the results of psychological experiments carried out to work out what increases and decreases willpower. Lots of those studies looked at how we deal with tempting foods! What Baumeister and Tierney conclude is that we each have a finite amount of willpower-energy each day and that it is used up making decisions and resisting temptations, so it gets depleted as the day goes by. No wonder evenings are so tricky for over-eating.

What replenishes willpower-energy is sleep and glucose. In other words, eating helps. Exactly what you're trying to avoid doing is what would give you more ability to avoid it. A Catch-22 if ever I heard one.

So, how do you deal with a challenging temptation when you've run out of your day's supply of willpower-energy?

Reduce the amount of willpower needed

You minimize the amount of willpower-energy you need at those tempting moments by having a ready-made simple but detailed plan to follow. You won't have the mental energy to come up with an effective plan at that point, so have one ready that you prepared earlier.

You'll need to rely on your Working Memory (see page 65) to put that plan into action. Creating a new habit is about the detail. Your new habit will be a very particular sequence of actions. Take the example of giving up biscuits with coffee at the office. If you haven't got a clear plan when the biscuit tin is being handed round, your brain will fixate its attention on the custard creams, and you'll have the mother of internal battles to come up with 'no thanks'. Instead, you need to have already run your brain through its paces so that it knows exactly what to do to get past the biscuit dilemma. We'll be looking at how to do this in the section on how to stop habitual eating (see page 191).

Just like Ronaldinho (see pages 93–4), you've got to do your thinking before you receive the ball. Then you just carry out the sequence you've already mentally practised. Declining biscuits, scoring international goals. The psychology is much the same.

The two-hand interweave technique

You also need a way of helping to deal with situations where you are on the verge of doing what you don't want to do (putting that snack in your mouth when you're not hungry or reaching for seconds). When you are about to do something out of line with your overall goal (the bigger picture of your goal), your brain is narrowly focusing in on the short-term reward.

Try this simple technique developed by Robin Shapiro (see page 277) to help resolve inner conflicts like this. It's called the two-hand interweave and it is thought to work by enhancing the communication between the left and right sides of your brain, allowing you to process the conflict. In effect this allows you to hold two options in mind and compare them.

Whenever you are at the nail-biting moment of 'Should I keep eating this meal or stop now?', imagine putting the positive choice (stop now) in one hand and the negative (keep eating) in the other. It doesn't matter which hand you use for which. Now open and close each hand alternately while you let your mind go back and forth between the two hands and just observe whatever happens. So you open your right hand and close your left, and then open your left and close your right, and keep alternating for a minute or so. Some people find this two-hand interweave really helps, and others don't. As with everything, you just need to fathom out what works for you.

There may be times when you still do the 'old' habit. If so, don't beat yourself up. Just remind yourself that this is just a blip and that you haven't fallen off any wagon. There's no need to abandon things for the rest of the day; just focus on planning what will be your next decision point.

How to resist pressure from others

Human beings are very social animals with a keen sense of social hierarchy. We constantly gauge our own status in relation to other people during social interactions, often unconsciously. We like to feel similar enough to other people to know we are playing the game correctly, but also like to feel better than others to know we are higher in the pecking order. We dislike situations in which we feel inferior.

In the modern Western world, being thin and eating less are attributes associated with higher status, while being overweight and eating more are associated with lower status. It is easy to feel that by eating food when someone else is declining food, you are sliding down the social scale bite by bite. If you're sharing a meal, it's reassuring to have the other person eating when you are, as it puts the two of you on a level at that moment. If one of you changes the script and eats less, it can feel threatening to the other person.

When you find yourself under pressure from others to eat more, the issue you are confronted with is separateness and autonomy. Others may want you to put food into your mouth to help them feel better. If you don't respond to this pressure by eating, their own lack of self-control may be exposed.

If this is happening to you, to lose weight you will need to move beyond merging with the crowd. You will need to use your own judgement about your own hunger and fullness based on the Appetite Pendulum™. Losing weight will involve shifting from using external triggers for eating, including other people's pressure, towards using internal signals. You can still eat with people, go out for meals and so on, but you won't eat as much as you used to and you won't eat when you're not hungry, usually. On the other hand, there may be times when you choose to eat dessert and they don't.

When you feel under pressure from other people around eating, remember:

» Others may want you to put food into your mouth to help them feel better. If you don't respond to this pressure by eating, their own lack of self-control may be exposed.

» When you find that someone close to you wants you to lose weight, this can be out of concern for your health, but all too often it is because they have their own issues around size and weight. A partner who does this may want you to get thin because they feel that your size somehow reflects on them negatively. Or the issue may be one of them wanting to control you.

» The pressure might be less overt from the other person and more about feeling a strong sense of competition, for instance with a sibling. Sibling rivalry is as old and as dangerous as Cain and Abel and as recent and newsworthy as Liam and Noel Gallagher.

» Your friend or relative may fear something else changing if you're successful. For example, that you'll leave them, or the group identity will be threatened. If you think this is the issue, then take your weight loss in gradual steps and see how it goes. Those close to you may need to see that other things don't change as the weight falls. They need time to adjust to your new weight, just as you do.

Samia described herself as a 'feeder' – she pushed food onto her children and anyone who visited her. Her biggest obstacle to losing weight was feeling under pressure socially to keep eating if others were still eating, even if she'd had enough. Eating around others had become fraught, and she wanted to change, but didn't know how without letting people close to her feel bad. We decided that her first step should be to stop pushing food onto people and instead, offer something once and restrain her urge to offer it again a few minutes later. Samia was to observe how people declined food and try using the phrases herself, such as 'That looks lovely but I won't have one just now thanks.' She also experimented with leaving a bit of food on her plate when eating out. It felt strange at first and one of her friends commented on the change, but that friend then told Samia she wanted to lose weight and the two agreed to support each other. Samia was pleasantly surprised to discover that she could act differently without causing her friends to feel bad.

In the next chapter you can learn about the five ways in which we eat when we are not hungry, any of which can prevent weight loss and lead us to keep gaining weight.

CHAPTER 7

Wait Until You're Definitely Hungry

Eating when you're not hungry is so common that most of my clients are puzzled when I ask them about it. Not about whether they eat when they aren't hungry, but whether they ever get hungry. For all sorts of reasons, we put food in our mouths without ever considering whether we are hungry. In developing Appetite Retraining, I've identified five types of non-hungry eating.

1. Habitual eating
2. Opportunistic eating
3. Insurance policy eating
4. Eating in response to cravings
5. Emotional eating

We'll look at these in more detail shortly. In each case, what's triggering eating involves your attention being captured by something other than what's happening in your gut.

When you're trying to lose weight, and tempted to eat when you're not hungry, you're in the situation of the kids subjected to the famous 'Marshmallow Test' by Walter Mischel, an eminent professor of psychology. A child is presented with a marshmallow and given a choice: eat this one now, or wait and enjoy two later. What will they do? It's a question of whether to go for immediate, smaller gratification or delayed, bigger reward. When you stop eating when not hungry you're shifting from the child who eats one now to the person who reaps the rewards later.

Benefits of waiting until you're definitely hungry

When you can pass on the biscuits being handed round, and deal with stress without eating, you can gain on several fronts. First and most immediately, by waiting to eat until you are definitely hungry, your next meal will taste fabulous because your taste buds will be at their most sensitive. By not eating all that extra, unnecessary food, you'll spend less money on replenishing the stores of the food you don't really want anyway. You will lose weight and the amount will depend on how much non-hungry eating you've been doing. You'll learn to be flexibly in control of your eating.

You can learn to wait until you're definitely hungry by using the Appetite Pendulum™ and the -3 rule (see opposite). Remember that if this is very different to what you do now, take this step by step so you move towards allowing yourself to feel definitely hungry by the next meal (or snack). If the thought of waiting to be definitely hungry makes you anxious, see page 211 'How to deal with anxiety'. Read that section now if you're feeling anxious just thinking about making this change.

The minus numbers on the Appetite Pendulum™ are the ones you tune in to between meals whenever you think of eating. The key to stopping non-hungry eating is to wait to eat until you are -3 (definitely hungry) on the scale.

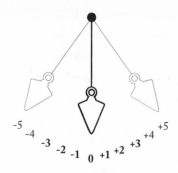

+5 uncomfortably full
+4 very full
+3 just full
+2 nearly full
+1 not sure, probably not hungry
 0 neutral
-1 not sure, probably a bit hungry
-2 slightly hungry
-3 definitely hungry
-4 very hungry
-5 extremely hungry

» −1 is a very slight feeling – you won't even notice it if you're busy doing something else.

» −2 starts to be noticeable with perhaps a slight tummy rumble.

» −3 is a definite feeling of hunger in your belly, perhaps with some rumbling sensations.

» −4 is starting to really intrude into your thinking – it will be hard to ignore thoughts about food, and you'll feel physically more uncomfortable in your belly, which will probably be growling more loudly.

» −5 is very uncomfortable and you'll find it hard not to think about food, as by then your brain is shouting at you, and you're likely to have gnawing sensations in your belly. You may start to feel faint. Once you are using Appetite Retraining correctly, you'll never hit -5 because you'll be in tune with your appetite.

'Whenever you think of eating, stop and ask yourself where you are on the Appetite Pendulum™ right now. If you aren't at -3, do anything – anything at all – except eat!'

As you retrain your appetite you are discovering what size and content of each meal allows you to keep going for a few hours until the next. The aim is to allow a bit of fat burning before each meal by getting definitely hungry by the time you eat, and as we've seen, this will not only aid your weight loss but will lead to other health benefits and make your next meal taste fantastic because of your taste bud sensitivity.

Between meals, whenever you think of eating, if you are not yet -3, but think you're -2 and it's less than an hour to your next meal, don't eat and instead distract yourself. The mild hunger will pass as your body will burn some fat and switch off the hunger signals for a while. By your mealtime you should then be -3 and you can really enjoy your lovely food. If you are at -2 and it's over an hour to your next meal, it would be wise to have a small snack to tide you over. If it's two hours or more, this snack will need to be something that keeps you going such as a few nuts or a banana. If it's somewhere between one and two hours until your next meal, try a snack that will be digested more quickly such as a handful of cherry tomatoes or a satsuma. You don't need to follow my snack suggestions if you'd prefer something else, but allow yourself to learn over the course of a few weeks which snack that you love will do the job of keeping you going for one to two hours, and which snack will keep you going for two to three hours. You're aiming to get to -3 by mealtimes because that means you're burning a bit of fat, but you don't want to get to -4 or -5 because you're more likely then to eat quickly and overeat, and less likely to really enjoy that meal.

The five types of non-hungry eating

Read on to learn more about how to stop the five types of non-hungry eating.

1. Habitual eating

In the 1890s, the Russian scientist Ivan Pavlov was studying salivation in dogs when he noticed that once they got used to a lab assistant giving them food, the dogs began to salivate when they saw the assistant come in to the lab, even when he didn't bring food. Curious to know more, Pavlov deliberately rang a bell every time food was presented and then found that ringing the bell on its own (with no food) produced salivation. Modern behavioural science was born.

Learning by association produces an expectation in us humans as well as dogs. And if what we expect is food, then our whole appetite system kicks in to operation and we start thinking about and wanting that food. Having biscuits with tea or salted nuts with wine can become a learned association whether we really fancy the snack at that point or not. How do you break associations which lead to the sort of mindless eating which is automatic but not really pleasurable, to make way for really lovely meals and snacks?

Because this sort of eating is automatic, you need to interrupt the automated sequence, bring it into Working

Memory and then deliberately perform a different action. Interrupting the automatic sequence is helped by putting an obstacle in its way, so that the automatic habit has to be re-set using your conscious mind. Remember my example of the teeth-brushing habit on page 66? The automated sequence of brushing your teeth swings into action at the sight of the toothbrush, and only falters if something in the sequence isn't right. An empty toothpaste tube means you have to re-engage your Working Memory and get a new tube out, so the sequence can resume.

With habitual non-hungry eating, you need to deliberately create this empty-toothpaste glitch so that you move from autopilot to deliberate Working-Memory control. The key is the interruption. For example, if you're trying to cut the tie between eating biscuits with a cup of tea, put the teabags or your mug somewhere odd, so that your tea-making sequence is altered. Or drink your tea from a handle-less cup or toughened glass so you need both hands to hold it and can't hold a biscuit so easily.

And at the point of being tempted to follow your old habit, ask yourself, 'Half an hour from now will I feel good that I ate this or good that I didn't?' so that you connect with the delayed gratification. It may strengthen your ability to wait.

If the trigger for your habitual eating is the time on the clock, ask yourself where you are right now on the Appetite Pendulum™. If you aren't definitely hungry, distract yourself with something fun or interesting. Text a friend to tell them you're resisting the biscuits, or look something up on the internet. Within minutes your focus will have gone past the snacking and you can get on with the next part of your day. You may find that simply recognizing that you've developed an unhelpful habit is enough. Remember, though, Appetite Retraining isn't about denying yourself: on days when you are hungry at tea break and really fancy a fabulous biscuit, have it. That is part of what joyful eating is all about.

Lourdes enjoyed a glass of wine in the evenings when watching TV, and was in the habit of having a bowl of crisps with it. The two things had become linked, so whenever she poured herself a glass of wine, she automatically reached for the crisps. Lourdes didn't want to give up the wine, but she did want to lose weight. Using the Appetite Pendulum™, she realized that she was still quite full from her evening meal so she decided to drop the bowl of crisps and focus instead on enjoying the wine and the TV programme. She put a note to herself on the door of the cupboard where the wine glasses were kept to remind herself of her weight loss goal so she would remember not to open the crisps cupboard. On the evenings when she felt restless without the snack, she did a Sudoku puzzle whilst watching the TV to distract herself from thoughts of crisps, which worked well for her.

---

2. Opportunistic eating

When you catch sight of food, the rest of the appetite system swings into action – brain, stomach, salivary glands. The whole shebang. All because that leftover cake was carelessly abandoned near your desk. It doesn't even have to be particularly appetizing to catch your eye. Who hasn't hoovered up someone else's buffet-lunch cast-offs?

How can you ignore food that just happens to be there, so that you can cut down on other people's leftovers and stop being a human recycling bin? And just eat what you really love, when your body is ready? What's likely to help most with cutting out opportunistic eating is altering your environment to remove the unhelpful food-cues. Put your treat foods in a high cupboard so that you have to get a stool or stretch a long way to reach them, or in a cupboard you rarely look in, so you don't get triggered to eat them by seeing them frequently. And at work, move any bowls of unhealthy foods further away from your desk, or put them in a cupboard you don't tend to look in.

If your opportunistic eating happens when you open the fridge, wrapping the unhealthy foods in opaque containers makes it easier not to eat them, and having pre-cut vegetables and fruit in see-through containers makes it much easier to snack on them. There's a definite theme here, which is that if you want to reduce opportunistic snacking, remove the food from your line of sight so your appetite doesn't get triggered. Or put an obstacle in the way, so you have to make an effort, which gives you valuable moments to change your mind.

If you work in catering and are surrounded by food continuously, opportunistic eating is more likely triggered than for the rest of us. How you handle this will depend on the particular environment you work in. If you're a chef and have to taste dishes frequently, perhaps you could decide that at work you'll get your nutrition for the day just through the tastings, which means eating more like grazing animals do. I know I said this isn't what we're built to do, and it's not, but in this situation, needs must. You could have small snacks in addition, perhaps fruit or vegetables, to balance the sauces you're tasting. That way, you're not tasting on top of three square meals a day – you're in effect replacing a meal with the tastings.

If you're another part of the restaurant team, you can work out your planned eating routine for working days around what the job allows. Then, use the combination of the Appetite Pendulum™ and the tips in this book to work out how to deal with the particular challenges in your place of work.

'Putting treats out of sight just makes it easier for you to avoid opportunistic eating.'

Lead us not into temptation!

Professor Brian Wansink has studied the effects of having food around the house or office on what we eat and his results are sobering reading. 'In sight, in stomach. We eat what we see, not what we don't.'

He found that women who had even one box of breakfast cereal visible anywhere in their kitchen weighed on average 9.5kg (21lb) more than their neighbour who didn't. Interestingly, people who had any fruit visible in a fruit bowl in the kitchen weighed on average 3kg (7lb) less than those who didn't. And when it comes to the office, people who had sweets on their desk ate twice as much as when the sweets were moved to six feet away.

Darcy sometimes put food on the table already plated up, and at other times put out bowls so people could serve themselves. She didn't find it difficult to stop at +3 when the meals were served on plates, as she had trained her eye to judge the quantity of food that would get her to feeling just full (+3), so it was easy to serve herself the right amount. But when the bowls were out on the table, she would keep picking from the bowls while chatting to her husband and often ended up at +4.

I suggested a couple of techniques to Darcy: first to put the bowls out of sight or, alternatively, put her own plate away and in its place, make a hot drink and keep it in front of her as something to focus on and enjoy, and to remind her to drink it rather than pick at the food in the bowls. Another suggestion was that she sits away from the table on an easy chair, so she can still chat with family after dinner but be out of reach of any food on the table.

---

3. Insurance policy eating

If you eat extra food now in case you're hungry later, it's like taking out an insurance policy against feeling hungry. Rather than risk hunger pangs, you take on extra food. But, remember, you already have an insurance policy: your stored fat. You need to cash this in a bit at a time by tolerating mild hunger.

How can you stop insurance policy eating? The solution is to learn to tolerate mild hunger. Once you can do this, you no longer need to eat excess in advance just in case – and this is part of the wonderful discovery that mild hunger is in fact your greatest ally when it comes to permanent weight loss.

First, whenever you're tempted to eat more now to avoid being hungry later, forget 'later'. Instead, ask yourself where you are on the Appetite Pendulum™ right now. If you're tempted to have a snack but aren't -3 (definitely hungry), then distract yourself. If you're thinking of eating a meal beyond the point of +3 (just full) in order to avoid being hungry later, don't. Stick to stopping at +3 and move on to doing something (anything) else away from food.

Second, remind yourself that getting hungry is allowing your body to burn some of your stored fat. When it does that, the hunger signals will go away again for a while (because your body registers the release of energy from the fat).

Tolerating mild hunger is mainly about how you handle the anxiety you feel about feeling hungry. If mild hunger makes you feel anxious, use one of the anxiety reduction strategies in Chapter 8. When you are tempted to eat in order to avoid getting hungry later, remind yourself that hunger is a sign that your body is starting to burn fat, so when you feel hungry it's a sign that you are actually losing weight. You will also notice that hunger comes and goes so that when you tolerate some mild hunger (-1 and -2 on the Appetite Pendulum™) it then subsides for a while.

4. Dealing with cravings

If I were a gambler, I'd bet my house on what you don't crave. I'd bet that you don't regularly crave healthy steamed vegetables, but I'm not that brave, or foolhardy. Let's just say that it's hugely more likely that you crave the sorts of things the supermarkets put at the checkouts that come in brightly coloured packets and have sugar, fat and salt high up on the ingredients list.

It's no accident that what you've got in your secret stash for those craving moments is a Snickers bar and tube of Pringles – not a bag of green beans. The Big Food manufacturers have studied your brain and know how to help it part with cash. Well, not your brain, but the brains and behaviours of people like you. What they know is that when they combine sugar, fat and salt in such a way as to produce a cascade of flavours and textures, the pleasure centre in your brain will go bananas. And the memory of that pleasure-frenzy will be etched in your mind together with a mental picture of the packaging. Next time you're in the queue, and you glimpse the packet out of the corner of your eye, the bliss-loaded memory trace is activated. Your appetite system swings into action. The Snickers bar is on the conveyor belt and Kerching! Mars notch up another sale.

How can you overcome cravings without eating?

Craving is a state of physical agitation, with a fixation on a specific food. In principle any of the anxiety-reducing strategies in Chapter 8 may help, so here I'll just describe one simple technique from Thought Field Therapy (TFT) developed by a Clinical Psychologist, Dr Roger Callahan, and described in his book *Tapping the Healer Within*.

TFT is a form of 'energy therapy', which applies some of the principles of acupressure tapping (acupuncture without the needles) to unpleasant emotional states. The essence of the approach is this: at the point of experiencing a craving, your body's energy system is in a state of imbalance. Introducing energy (by tapping on specific points on the body in a particular sequence) can correct this. To reduce the urge to eat:

1. Think of the food you're craving, as vividly as possible.
2. Rate your urge for that food on a 0–10 scale where 0 is no urge at all and 10 is really intense.

3. While focusing on the thought of the food you crave, take two fingers of one hand and tap 10 times under the eye, about an inch below the bottom of the centre of the bony orbit, high on the cheek.

4. Tap solidly 10 times under the arm, about four inches below the armpit.

5. Tap the 'collarbone' point 10 times. To locate it, find the U-shaped bone at the base of your throat (where the knot of a man's tie would sit), then move down an inch and to the right one inch. This is the collarbone point.

6. Now rate the urge again on the 0–10 scale. If you no longer feel the craving, you can get on with your day.

There are other steps to Dr Callahan's urge reduction which you can find out more from his website (see page 283). I've found TFT helps many people, but not all.

If TFT isn't doing anything for your craving, experiment with the other anxiety reduction techniques in Chapter 8 when you get a craving. You may need to ban the foods you crave from your home, at least while you learn how to deal with them. Once you no longer crave them you probably won't want to buy them. Instead you can discover which fabulous food really hits the spot for you when you really fancy something sweet or salty. I suggest you do keep that fabulous food at home, or buy it just for special occasions, in small portion sizes. Ignore the 3 for 2 offers and just buy the amount you will have for your next fabulous treat. If it's something that keeps well, have it in a cupboard out of sight. If it can be frozen, it can obviously sit in the freezer. If it's something that can't be kept, try to buy it only for special planned times.

Carys struggled to eat just one piece of cake. She found that despite trying to avoid sweet foods, she would often give in to a craving for cake in the afternoon or evening and then couldn't stop eating it. It made her feel weak and hopeless about getting more control over her eating. She was in a pattern of bingeing on sweet foods and desperate to break out of it.

We did two things to reduce the amount of cake she was eating, without reducing the pleasure she got from it. First, we planned two particularly lovely treats into her day: a latte coffee with sugar mid-afternoon and a single piece of cake at 9pm. Second, she learned the TFT tapping technique (see page 199). Whenever Carys had a craving from now on, she was to use the tapping technique while remembering that she could look forward to the afternoon latte (if she had cravings in the afternoon) and could look forward to the evening cake (if she had cravings in the evening). Within a few weeks, Carys established this new pattern and found that some days she didn't want the latte or the cake, but she always knew she could have it if she wanted. Her sugar consumption dropped dramatically as a result of the combination of having planned treats and using the tapping technique.

Emotional eating

Stress, boredom and sadness, amongst other emotional states, easily become tied up with eating. We are naturally wired to move away from pain and towards pleasure, and when we encounter pain (physical or emotional), we strive to get away from it. Food naturally activates the pleasure systems in the brain; some foods more effectively than others. So in the presence of a painful emotion, one option is to self-medicate using food.

Emotional eating is such a big issue that I've devoted a whole chapter to it. Chapter 8 explains that our emotions are a wordless language that our body uses to tell us what is going on inside us and around us. If you don't understand the language, and always respond to painful feelings by eating, you may mask the feeling but find yourself in a repeating cycle:

feel it

˅

stuff it down with food

˅

mask it

As you'll see in Chapter 8, you can learn to decipher what those difficult emotions are telling you, and discover how to respond without using food. You'll find that the feelings can be managed. As you lose the emotional-eating weight you've carried, you'll feel stronger and more confident than before.

'When you slip up and eat something when you aren't hungry, make a note of how satisfying (or not) it was. Repeatedly realizing how disappointing these non-hungry eating sessions are can help when you're next tempted.'

CHAPTER 8

—

Stop Emotional Eating

Emotions are our body and brain's way of telling us what is happening to us. They are essential for our physical and social survival. Our emotions are like an internal non-verbal language and each one has a particular message, like our body communicating with our brain via an ancient code. For instance, sadness tells us we've lost something important to us, whereas fear tells us we're in danger.

Emotions also have a communicative function in that our facial expressions and actions can show other people what we feel. But what we're concerned with here is the internal, private face of emotions. Emotional eating means eating in response to emotional states rather than because we are physically hungry. When you are physically hungry, it's food that you need to satisfy the hunger, but when you're eating because you feel sad, angry or anxious, the food will never really satisfy you.

Here we'll look at how not to eat for emotional reasons, so that eating is a pleasure you can really enjoy when you eat because you're hungry, and so that you don't eat unnecessary, unpleasurable and unhealthy foods when your body doesn't need them.

'Your self-confidence will grow as you learn how to manage difficult feelings.'

Physical versus emotional hunger

Put simply, physical hunger is when your Appetite Pendulum™ number is between -1 and -5 (see page 189). There are degrees of physical hunger from very slight hunger (-1) to feeling extremely hungry (-5). The better you get at gauging where you are on the Appetite Pendulum™, the easier it will be to distinguish physical and emotional hunger.

Of course, you might have both types of hunger (physical and emotional) at the same time. In which case, it will help you to eat what resonates with you (see Chapter 9 for more on this) and just have the amount you've learned your body needs. In addition, it will help to identify what feeling you are experiencing from those covered in this chapter and use the suggestions to deal with the feeling directly.

Why do we eat for emotional reasons?

Emotional comfort and eating are entwined from the baby's first feed. The closeness and warmth associated with being held and fed are all part of the same nutritional and emotional nourishment. Some of us return to food for comfort more than others later in life and we come to associate food with easing distressing emotions. People often reward children with 'treat' food when they've done something good, or to ease pain and distress when they are hurt. This isn't inherently wrong, but it's helpful to recognize that if a parent always responds to a child's different emotions by giving them sweet or salty foods, then the child will associate those foods with soothing those emotional states and will turn to them without thinking when they face emotional pain. It may also mean that the child doesn't distinguish between different emotional states and so may not realize when they are angry as opposed to anxious.

As I mentioned in Chapter 2, your appetite system has links to the pleasure centres in the brain and to the part of the brain that deals with fear. Food can affect both of these systems, and you may have found that eating takes the edge off difficult feelings or even numbs them. It's likely that some foods work better than others and modern manufactured foods are in some ways like extremely cheap drugs, at least for some of us. And you don't need a prescription to get hold of them.

I'll go through the main things that drive emotional eating now, and give you some easy-to-follow advice about how to deal with each emotion directly, without going to the kitchen. We'll take each emotion in turn, look at what its coded message is, and how you can respond to each emotion without reaching for food.

Ramon's senior job in a multi-national company was stressful. He had developed heart problems and his doctor had told him to lose weight and cut down on alcohol. Ramon said that when he was alone, either away on business or at home, he would eat due to boredom and stress. His was a classic example of emotional eating – he found that food somehow numbed the stress and eating alleviated the boredom. But this had adverse effects on his health– weight gain and heart problems – and it affected his confidence.

Ramon found that using an Anxiety Release App (see page 214) was very effective in reducing his stress levels at the end of the day, and he would go for a short brisk walk if he had any remaining feelings of stress. Walking while listening to the App soon became a regular habit as it worked so well for him. Having an alternative way of dealing with stress instead of eating made Ramon better about himself. To deal with the boredom, he bought a MENSA quiz book and started doing online shopping or playing computer games when he was on his own. We agreed that he would plan a fabulous late evening savoury snack to look forward to – he chose his favourite: pickles and strong cheese. Ramon lost 13kg (28lb) in five months by changing this emotional eating pattern.

How to deal with anxiety

Fear is our body's way of telling us that we are in danger. Anxiety is the feeling we experience when there is no immediate danger but we feel afraid. This happens when some sort of threat is detected, even though the threat isn't real, because the brain uses the better-safe-than-sorry principle where potential threats are concerned.

You are anxious if:

» You feel fearful and threatened in the absence of physical danger.
» You have physical sensations such as shortness of breath, increased heart rate, nausea, sweating and trembling.

These physical sensations occur because the body enters a state of 'fight or flight' as a surge of adrenaline is released. The heart pumps harder and breathing gets faster to supply the muscles with extra oxygen to run away or fight the threat. But if there isn't actually a threat, what do you do with these unnecessary and uncomfortable sensations? There are several ways to handle them – try a few to discover which works best for you.

1. Steady Breathing

One of the physical changes produced by the adrenaline surge is faster, shallower breathing. Mostly breathing is automatic, but we can deliberately change the depth and speed of the breaths we take, which means that we can change our breathing pattern back to the non-anxious one.

Focus on the breath coming in and out of your lungs. Put your left hand on your chest and your right hand on your belly. When you are anxious your breathing may be all where your left hand is, shallow and tight. Move the centre of your breathing down towards your belly by making the in-breath a bit slower and deeper. Inhale slowly and deeply through your nose while you count to five. Then release the breath gently and slowly through your mouth. Notice that your breathing is now reaching deeper, where your right hand is resting. Keep breathing like this until you feel the anxiety has gone. This is known as 'diaphragmatic breathing'.

2. Calm Place Visualization

This is the 'Safe Place' technique developed by Dr Francine Shapiro, described in her book *Getting Past Your Past*. Here we are using Dr Shapiro's visualization technique to access feelings of calm. You cannot feel calm and anxious at the same time, so using your conscious mind to access a calm image can help reduce the anxious feelings.

First, think of a place you associate with being calm. It could be somewhere you have been on holiday, or somewhere in nature or on a favourite journey. Bring this calm place to mind. Imagine yourself being there. Close your eyes if this helps. Use your mind's eye to look around and notice what you can see in this place. What time of day would you most like it to be? What would you choose the weather to be like? Take in the most pleasing and calming visual elements of this scene. Now notice what sounds there are, particularly the sounds that are relaxing to you. Also notice what smells you associate with this place and really tune into these. Finally, in this calm place, are you standing, sitting or lying down? Notice the feel of whatever you are standing, sitting or lying on and feel the sensations of your body against it. If you are sitting or lying down, allow your body to relax a bit more and notice how relaxed you feel in this place. If you are standing or walking, notice the ground beneath your feet and the sensations of your feet on the ground. Notice how grounded and calm you feel. Bring this calm place to mind whenever you feel anxious.

3. Bilateral stimulation

Bilateral stimulation means alternate stimulation to left and right sides of the body or brain. Our brains are made up of two separate but connected hemispheres, left and right. Because of how our brain-body connections work, bilateral stimulation of the body produces bilateral stimulation of the two brain hemispheres. Research shows that bilateral stimulation of the brain can be very effective in reducing feelings of anxiety.

Bilateral stimulation can be achieved through tapping on the left and right side of your body alternately at a rate of about one left-then-right pair of taps per second, or listening to tones presented to left and right ears alternately. Mark Grant, a Clinical Psychologist has produced an App called 'Anxiety Release with Bilateral Stimulation' (see page 283). There are five tracks on this, including the Safe Place visualization described above. In order to get the helpful effect of the alternating tones, you need to listen to the App through headphones.

4. Positive Self-Talk

How we talk to ourselves silently in our heads has a significant bearing on how we feel and how our bodies react. This is what Cognitive Therapy, one of the most widely used and well-researched forms of psychological therapy, is based on. Using positive, realistic ways of talking to yourself can significantly alter how you experience anxiety and significantly reduce it. 'Realistic' is important here. Cognitive Therapy does not involve overly positive or unrealistic self-talk as it does not work.

A simple example would be, 'This is a wave of anxiety. It is unpleasant but not dangerous. I can ride the wave of anxiety or use breathing or tapping to reduce it.'

Eleanor had grown up in a family where emotional expression was discouraged. She had internalized the view that to show feelings is a 'bad thing' and had never learned how to regulate her emotions without using food. She had discovered as a child that when she felt bad, she could make herself feel better by eating sweets or biscuits, and this naturally became her emotional coping mechanism. Eleanor was aware that she often felt anxious in work meetings, so I began by teaching her techniques to reduce her anxiety. She found diaphragmatic breathing and TFT tapping both helped, and she was soon much more able to respond to feeling anxious by breathing or tapping. Eleanor began to see emotions as something to be accepted and understood rather than pushed away.

How to deal with worrying

Worrying about something is your brain's way of telling you that there is something unresolved in your mind that you need to attend to. There are two different types of worrying, productive and unproductive. Productive worrying refers to something that you can do something about. Acknowledging that there is a problem and deciding to tackle it can stop the worry. For a productive worry you can take practical steps to help resolve the problem. Problem-solving involves defining the problem precisely, brain-storming as many alternative solutions as you can, choosing which of the brain-storm options looks most promising, putting it into action and if it doesn't work choosing the next most likely looking option.

On the other hand, if the worry is about something that can't be dealt with in this way, it is an 'unproductive worry'. Allocating 'worry time', such as 4pm each day, to the issue can help, then, when that time comes, put a timer on for 15 minutes and think about the worrying issue then, and keep focused on it, maybe writing notes. When the timer goes off, put the notes away and leave any further thinking about it until the worry time the following day. This way, when the worry pops into your mind at other times you think, 'I don't need to think about that now as I have made time for it later.' The most helpful thing you can do with an unproductive worry is to realize that it's not solvable, and that whatever it is has to be accepted as something out of your control.

How to deal with boredom

Boredom is our body's way of telling us that we are under-stimulated. People vary in how much stimulation they need to keep their nervous system operating at an optimal level. Some people have an already-reactive nervous system and need relatively little additional stimulation from the outside world to feel comfortable; indeed, they may get over-stimulated easily and need to retreat from further stimulation. Some people, on the other hand, have a less reactive nervous system and need much more external stimulation to keep sufficiently stimulated to feel comfortable, so tend to be more sensation-seeking. If you are a sensation-seeking type of person in an un-stimulating environment, you will feel restless. You may have found that food gives you some stimulation at these times, so is better than nothing, but you may well then keep eating because it isn't enough, or the right sort of stimulation.

Allow the possibility that the bored, restless feeling is trying to tell you something. Don't try to squash or ignore it. Listen to it and start to notice what 'part' or aspect of yourself is feeling bored. It is probably the part that needs stimulation and variety. You may have developed a pattern of feeding it with tasty food. That is fine if you are physically hungry at the time. If you aren't physically hungry, eating tasty food will not do the trick and you will still feel restless. Look for other sources of stimulation and try one when you next get that boredom-hunger feeling. It could be a hobby or interest, a puzzle or surfing the internet.

Debbie tended to eat when she was bored and exhausted at the end of a working day, so she explored other ways of using very low-energy activities to simultaneously stimulate and calm her. She found that what did the trick for her was surfing the internet looking at interior design sites as she loved soft furnishings and home design. She didn't have enough energy on workday evenings to actually make anything, but looking for inspiration and ideas on the internet was a great alternative.

'You may need different distractions at times of day. For example, when you're tired you'll need some low-energy distractions such as doing a puzzle, surfing the internet, doing a relaxing craft activity, reading or watching TV. When you're feeling more energetic, you could garden, exercise, do chores or learn a new language for distraction.'

How to deal with stress

Stress is your body's way of telling you you're over-stimulated. This highly aversive state tends to lead to feelings of agitation and will lead to you urgently seeking things to take the stimulation levels back to a comfortable range.

Each of us has a comfortable range for our nervous system activation – anything above that is aversive and makes us stressed. Anything below our comfortable range is also unpleasant and we feel bored, as we've seen.

If you eat in response to stress, it is probably because you have learned to associate eating with feeling calmer, but any amount of food will only numb the stressed feelings. The key to dealing with stress is to reduce your nervous system's over-stimulation. You may find that calming activities help, but you may be surprised to find that other sorts of stimulation (such as dancing to loud music) help to discharge the over-stimulated state and return you to your comfortable range. The key here is to find activities that calm your over-stimulated nervous system.

As you build your resources and learn to react to stress without eating, your perception of yourself is likely to shift towards recognizing strengths you may not have been aware of. As this happens you may find that you can start to reduce the external stresses on you further by taking active steps to change your circumstances or developing the confidence to deal with (or distance yourself from) people who are causing you stress.

Jemma's most stressful time of day was the drive home from collecting her children from school and the stress stayed high right up until bathtime. Jemma was a high-flyer at work, but when she got behind the wheel to drive home, her nerves started jangling. Just the anticipation of her kids arguing and whining in the back was enough to make a detour to the petrol station to stock up on chocolate, to calm her before she got to the school gates. On arriving home, she'd simultaneously cook tea whilst attempting to oversee homework, and she was so busy that she couldn't stop and stand back to see the bigger picture.

When we looked at this together, the first thing Jemma realized was that her children's bad temperedness in the car could be because they were hungry and tired. So she tried making up a healthy snack for each of them in a Tupperware box for the next day. Then when she picked them up, she handed each child their snack and they happily ate it on the way home. The tension eased noticeably.

Next, Jemma made up her own little Tupperware with a few olives and cubes of feta cheese – a favourite of hers. Instead of pulling into the petrol station, Jemma chose a nice spot on the road between work and school and sat for a couple of minutes enjoying her own lovely snack. With things calmer all round, Jemma realized that her children were at an age where she didn't need to supervise their homework. If they didn't do it, they'd have to face the teacher themselves and explain.

Simple practical tweaks to her day meant that Jemma's stress levels reduced dramatically, her energy levels increased and she lost half a stone in a few weeks of this small change to dealing with the most stressful part of her day.

How to deal with sadness

Feelings of sadness are about loss or absence. They are your body's way of telling you that you have lost something important to you. When we suffer a loss, it creates an emotional injury; the emotional equivalent of a physical injury. Your brain can heal, just as your body can heal, although when it's a major loss you don't always go back to being completely how you were before. To help it heal, try doing things that will protect the emotional injury while it heals. Be gentle with it. Normal sadness is a temporary feeling and can be helped by acknowledging the feeling to yourself and allowing yourself or someone else to take care of you until the feeling passes.

Self-care includes:

» Being compassionate and easy towards yourself
» Remembering that the feeling will pass
» Soothing your senses using music, gentle lighting, pleasant smells and comfortable clothes
» Spending time on an undemanding and soothing pastime, perhaps watching a film, going for a walk or having a bath

A particular type of sadness is feeling lonely. If you feel lonely, then it's likely that contact with someone would be helpful, which could be by phone, or text if you aren't able to be with someone in person.

How to deal with anger

Anger is our body's way of telling us we have been wronged or hurt. It produces sensations of hot displeasure and feelings of hostility and a desire for retaliation.

Eating in response to feeling angry can feel like stuffing the anger back inside rather than letting it out. It can help numb the feelings but has the side-effect of weight gain. Dealing with anger directly means finding a way of discharging the intense feelings it produces. The following can help to discharge such feelings:

» Tell the person who has caused the anger what you think, or visualize doing this

» Do some physical exercise

» Listen to loud, aggressive or uplifting music

» Write down your thoughts and feelings and then destroy what you have written

» Channel the anger into a productive or creative activity, such as painting, writing or pottery

» Use energy psychology techniques such as the anger sequence from TFT (see page 283)

How to deal with guilt

Guilt is our body and brain's way of telling us we have transgressed a rule or moral principle that's important to us. Two types of guilt are relevant here.

The first is when you eat in response to feelings of guilt about something you have done or have failed to do. As with any other emotional eating, the food may numb the feeling or distract you but it does not effectively deal with the feeling. In fact, the feeling is likely to pop up again, at which point you will eat again and so the cycle continues.

Dealing with guilt effectively involves scrutinizing what you did and deciding what if anything you need to do about it. To deal with guilt, ask yourself:

» Exactly what have I done that was wrong or sinful?
» Who exactly did this hurt?
» What reparation do I need to make to this person?
» What law or rule have I broken?
» What penalty do I need to pay?
» If I can't repair the damage or pay the penalty, what can I learn from this experience?
» Do I need to change my view of myself to assimilate and accept what I have done? (For example, being able to see yourself as someone who has done something they regret.)

Guilt can get in the way of being able to look after yourself if you don't feel deserving, but the part of you that feels the pain of the guilt is a vulnerable part and it hurts so much because of how hard it is to bear hurting someone else. You feel the guilt because you're a good person, not because you're bad.

The second type of guilt arises in relation to eating. In relation to food, the only reason food might be bad is if it makes you ill. Unfortunately, modern dieting has encouraged a mind-set of seeing some foods as bad and others as good and people then feel guilty about eating the 'bad' ones. Food you really like isn't bad; it's lovely, it's a blessing.

In *French Women Don't Get Fat* Mireille Giuliano says that the influence of Anglo-Saxon Protestantism led eating and other pleasures to be sinful and therefore guilt-ridden. Giuliano points out that if you buy in to this view of pleasurable food being sinful, you're likely to feel bad when you eat it. You can't enjoy it fully because it's 'naughty', but as she says, many of us who think like this blatantly eat far too much of it. She contrasts this with people who can see pleasurable food as joyful, eat it and really savour it, but then stop eating and enjoy (rather than regret) the fact that they have eaten something they have really enjoyed.

The other issue with guilt and eating is not being able to do something good for yourself. Over the years I have seen very many people who equate looking after themselves with selfishness and badness. Many of those people arrive in my consulting room depleted and exhausted, often on anti-depressants. What they struggle to comprehend is that the more you deplete yourself, the less you are able to help people who rely on you. The more you nourish yourself with good food and self-care, the more energy and resources you have to help others. If you don't believe me, try it for a week. Suspend your disbelief that I might be right and make a point of eating food you love and resting when you can and doing as much as possible to restore and recharge your batteries. Then notice how much you are willing and able to do for other people.

> **'As with any other emotional eating, the food may numb the feeling or distract you but it does not effectively deal with the feeling. In fact, the feeling is likely to pop up again, at which point you will eat again and so the cycle continues.'**

How to deal with happiness

Food has been tied up with celebration since time immemorial. Eating together strengthens bonds. There is absolutely no problem about food being a focus of celebration and joy. The reason it's in this chapter is that many people I've worked with say their emotional overeating takes place through rewarding themselves when things go well.

If you are using food to reward yourself too much, so that you're lining up the treats at the end of every working day, it will help if you can broaden your range of 'rewards'. It can still be 'naughty but nice' if that's what you're after, like a trashy novel, a favourite box set or a candle-lit bubble bath. It will be fun to think up what your alternative (calorie-free) guilty pleasure is going to be. Then you can keep the family size box of chocolates for when there are other people to enjoy them with and make an occasion of it.

Having one special fabulous snack in the evening rather than many mediocre snacks may help you to reward yourself without overeating. The trick here is to work out what time is the best for you to really enjoy the snack, and to structure the rest of your evening around it. A snack that is looked forward to like this can make it easier to structure your evenings, and to think 'I'll wait for my fabulous snack.'

For example, you might want to have it at 8.30pm, which would mean being able to look forward to it, and reminding yourself that before that time you'll distract yourself away from food if you're tempted. Brushing your teeth after your lovely snack and having a hot drink can help you stop eating more afterwards.

A note on overwhelming emotions

Most of us have at some time experienced feelings that were so intense that we weren't sure how we could keep going. But for some people, extremely intense emotions are a regular occurrence and make day-to-day life very difficult. This can happen following traumatic experiences where the trauma remains very much present in the mind. Being repeatedly overwhelmed by re-experiencing flashbacks to a trauma means that you are experiencing post-traumatic stress and you may need further help (see Resources, page 275).

Overwhelming emotions are also a feature of Borderline Personality Disorder (or Emotionally Unstable Personality Disorder), which itself is often related to previous trauma. If you've been diagnosed with Borderline Personality Disorder, the intensity of the feelings is likely to need additional techniques to the ones in this chapter. More information about dealing with intense emotional states is given in the Resources section on pages 277 and pages 278–9.

As you retrain your appetite to eat only when hungry and stop eating when you're just full, you'll be eating less than you did before. Which means that what you eat is more important than ever – you want your smaller meals to be as delicious, joyful and satisfying as possible. So in the next chapter we'll look at how to know what to eat. This is not about following someone else's list of permitted foods; it's about learning to tune in to what your body wants and needs.

CHAPTER 9

—

Know What to Eat

If you've tried dieting before, you may be struggling to know what to eat. 'Diet-think' is the confusing state of knowing lots of rules, but not knowing which are worth following, like a game of nutritional Quidditch. Nutritional information in the media is utterly confusing and it's hard to know who to listen to. Super-foods, clean-eating, low-carb, low-fat, high-fat, paleo. The list is long. The more you try to follow specific nutritional rules, the further you get from really listening to your body. And that's a shame, because when you tune in to your hunger signals, you can start to 'hear' what your body actually wants.

And what your body wants is not that tube of Pringles. Well, not often. It's real food. When you're actually hungry, your taste buds are buzzing and real food tastes great. But if you're not hungry your taste bud sensitivity is dulled, so you'll need high sugar, high fat, high salt combinations to be able to taste anything much at all.

In this chapter we'll look at how to listen to your body to discern what to eat when you are hungry, so that you can stop grazing through the contents of your fridge in search of something you just can't seem to find. And we'll see that when you listen to your body, the range of foods you eat will become more balanced.

Listening to your gut

According to the authors of *The Psychologist's Eat-Anything Diet*, Leonard and Lillian Pearson, one of the most common causes of overeating is that people don't eat enough of what they love. It is easier to stop eating when you are eating food you love because it satisfies your appetite for pleasure. You feel good, sooner. Maximizing pleasure happens when you eat when you are definitely hungry, by tuning in to the messages from your body signalling what you are hungry for right now and choosing that food.

A common mistake is to choose foods that tempt you because you see or smell them, without tuning in to whether it is that food you have an appetite for right now.

Another common mistake is to ignore your body's signals and instead rely on what you think you want. Often this results in people turning to sweet or salty foods because they think of them as treats and the thinking goes something like, 'I love chocolate so I will really enjoy chocolate now.' If your body really wants something different, you will feel dissatisfied even after you have eaten the chocolate and may eat more of it to try to attain the feeling of satisfaction. There is a way to avoid this happening.

As you become more attuned to your gut to tell you when you are hungry, you will find that it signals not just when to eat but also what type of food, whether sweet or savoury, and perhaps which particular sweet or savoury. These signals are subtler and you may not come up with specifically what you want to eat, but they can guide you in which type of food is most appealing right now.

Once you are hungry, some foods will hit the spot and some won't. When you are eating the wrong thing it won't feel satisfying, even if you thought it is what you wanted. This section is to help you learn how to predict what food will hit the spot so you don't find yourself half way through a cake, wishing that you'd chosen a Spanish omelette.

This is why what you have in your cupboards and fridge should be foods you like, not what you think you should have. It's only the foods you really like that will ever really hit the spot. If you have been following diets that tell you what foods to eat, you may have absorbed an idea of what you 'should' be eating to lose weight. Put that aside. Ban 'diet foods' from your life. Instead, start tuning in to your gut to hear what your body wants to eat instead of listening to diets, the food industry or anyone else.

'If your body really wants something different, you will feel dissatisfied even after you have eaten the chocolate and may eat more of it to try to attain the feeling of satisfaction. There is a way to avoid this happening.'

Food groups

As omnivores we can eat a wide range of foods. We each have preferences for particular foods. Foods are grouped in the chart according to type:

Protein	Fish, seafood, poultry, meat, soya, eggs, beans, pulses, nuts, seeds
Carbohydrate	Whole grains, beans, pulses, potatoes, rice, pasta, bread, fruit, vegetables, dairy
Fats	Seeds, nuts, avocados, oily fish, oils, butter

You will no doubt recognize these foods as those that are generally seen as part of a balanced diet, although some weight-loss diets work by excluding or restricting certain food groups.

Sweet foods	Cakes, biscuits, chocolate, sweets, desserts, ice cream, fizzy drinks and other sweet foods
Savoury foods	Crisps, salted nuts, salty snacks, ketchup, mayonnaise and other salty and fatty foods

You will be aware that these are foods that are not necessary to sustain life, but which are tasty and appetizing and can give us genuine pleasure. With Appetite Retraining instead of banning these foods, they are welcomed as part of varied 21st-century food choices. The point is that the genie is out of the bottle in relation to salt and sugar. Many of us who have tasted delicious desserts or tasty savouries like them and we know that they exist. Indeed, we are reminded of them daily through advertising and widespread availability.

Your favourite foods exercise

Now for the exercise:

Step 1: Identify your favourite foods

Write down your favourite foods. They can be any sort of food – something as simple as a single raw item (e.g. a peach) or as complicated as a cooked dish (e.g. chicken Kiev). Be honest about this, and allow yourself to take time to compile the list.

Put the favourite foods in the relevant groups (see page 236). Some foods may fit more than one group so just put them in the group that seems to fit best. For example, chicken Kiev would go in the protein group as the main part of it is chicken. Spaghetti bolognese on the other hand could be included in both protein and carbohydrates because it's a portion of pasta with a portion of bolognese. Now look at your list: are there foods in each of the carbohydrate, protein and fat categories? Does your list include any fresh fruit and vegetables? If there is a balance, great. These are the foods that you will eat from now on. Go and buy those and have some of them available. Now that you have learned to use your gut to tell you when to start and when to stop eating, these foods are the ones you will want to eat when you are hungry.

If your list is not varied, let's look at what you are missing. For a list that does not include certain types of food (carbohydrate, protein, fats), identify what your favourite foods are in those categories so you can add them. If you need to follow a low-carbohydrate plan, focus on which carbs you like best. There is increasing interest in low-carbohydrate eating among some doctors and researchers, particularly for people who are diabetic or are insulin-resistant. I'm not qualified to comment on this, but you can find out more in Michael Mosley's *8-Week Blood Sugar Diet*.

If you do not like any food in a particular category, you can educate your taste buds, although if you have no foods in the 'Sweet foods' or 'Savoury foods' categories there is no need to expand your diet to include these.

If all your favourite foods are sugary or fatty, you may have become hooked on these foods, perhaps because of eating when you're not hungry and needing the heightened saltiness or sweetness to taste much at all. Developing your ability to wait to eat until hungry will help with this, as will dealing with cravings (see page 198) for these particular processed foods.

Step 2: Expand your range of favourite foods

Discovering new foods is joyful in itself, and increasing the range of foods you eat can bring additional health benefits. Professor Tim Spector's research on the microbiome in our gut (the population of different strains of micro-organisms) has revealed the health benefits of being adventurous with what we eat because the wider the range of foods we eat, the more species of bacteria we have in our gut, and this variety is good for our health and may make losing weight easier.

Try tasting one new food each week to see which you like. To expand your range of favourite fruits, try eating one new fruit each week until you have tried everything available. As well as fresh fruit, try dried, frozen and tinned fruits. The same principle applies to vegetables – try new types of vegetables as well as those in jars and tinned and frozen vegetables.

You can repeat this exercise with different types of bread to find the ones you like best. As the amount of food you are now eating will be less than before, you could try more expensive breads.

The same applies to expanding your range of protein. Try out different ways of cooking meat, fish, pulses etc or buying different ready-prepared versions and try new ones when eating out. If you want to increase the range of dairy food you eat, try tasting different cheeses and yoghurts.

You may find that you like foods from different countries and cultures, which are more widely available than ever.

Any new foods you really like will be part of what you eat from now on. Anything you don't like, forget about. The favourite foods exercise will take time, so don't wait to do the next step (going shopping) until you've completed it.

'Try tasting one new food each week to see which you like.'

Going food shopping

Food shopping covers meals and snacks and from now on your trolley should be full of things you love. Whether you cook from scratch (often better from a taste point of view if you have time) will depend on your lifestyle and cooking skills. Meal ingredients or ready meals should be chosen on the basis of what you (and anyone you cook for) enjoy.

Snacks should also be things that you love, and it may help to have a few different types of things in the house for times when you need a snack to keep you going. Think about getting a range of snacks that will keep you going for different amounts of time. For example, a handful of cherry tomatoes will satisfy your hunger for a much shorter time than a few nuts.

And when you are thinking about the sweet or salty foods categories, make sure that what you choose is something you really love, in the right quantity for a meal or snack. Given how large a lot of 'individual' portions are now, one 'portion' will probably do you for two different meal or snack times. In which case it may be best to halve it and freeze half as soon as you get home.

The issue of portion sizes is central to Appetite Retraining and when you shop, you need to think in terms of how much food will get you to +3, not what food will be the cheapest per gram. There is evidence that when we buy food in smaller-sized packages, we eat less. So a multipack of bags of crisps is going to be easier to eat in moderation than a family-pack that once opened, may be difficult to put away. If you eat the whole family pack, not only have you eaten way more than you need, but it has also cost more.

By the same token, you'll need to think about BOGOF and 3-for-2 type offers in a different light. These offers are great if they are for tins with a long shelf life, which will mean real value, but if it's something with a looming use-by date, be honest with yourself… you'll probably eat it all by then to avoid 'waste'. See page 105 for more of my rant on waste.

The other thing to steer clear of is foods that you find 'addictive'. I mean anything that, if it's in the house, you won't rest until it's all gone. Save that food for when you no longer have that compulsive reaction to having it nearby.

By the end of your shopping trip you should have in your house a small range of things you love. Don't buy foods you don't like but think you should eat because they are 'healthy', and foods you find you only binge on.

> 'There is evidence that when we buy food
> in smaller-sized packages, we eat less. So
> a multipack of bags of crips is going to be
> easier to eat in moderation than a family-
> pack that once opened, may be difficult
> to put away.'

Crockery and cutlery

There's a new academic discipline called 'neurogastronomy', which studies the complex brain mechanisms that give rise to flavour perception, and which has been publicized by Heston Blumenthal, the Michelin-starred-chef-cum-chemistry-professor. Neurogastronomist Professor Charles Spence's book *Gastrophysics: The New Science of Eating* outlines all sorts of influences on our enjoyment of food beyond the taste.

The weight of the knives and forks we use influences our enjoyment of a meal – food is judged to be of higher quality when eaten using heavy cutlery. Crockery makes a difference too. If you hold the bowl you are eating from in one hand and your spoon or fork in the other, the weight in your hand will make you feel more satisfied with whatever amount you eat. A study used three bowls of differing weights filled with the same amount of yoghurt. When people held the bowl in their hand while eating, the yoghurt in the heaviest bowl was rated as having a more intense flavour and being more expensive, and was more liked than that from the lightest bowl, even though the three bowls contained the same yoghurt.

In another study, strawberry desserts were rated as 10 per cent sweeter and 15 per cent more flavourful when eaten from a white plate compared with black plate, so that is a simple thing to buy if you want extra sweetness without adding extra calories. And if you drink from a heavier glass, you get more satisfaction from the same drink. These are simple ways to enhance your enjoyment without increasing your portion size.

Gauging what you're hungry for right now

What you're hungry for when you are definitely hungry (-3 on the Appetite Pendulum™) is going to be food that you already love, or a new delicious discovery. And when you do feel definitely but not overly hungry, not all foods will appeal to you equally. Unlike if you are completely ravenous, at which point you may not care what you eat, as long as you eat something. And, as we've seen before, when you're that hungry, you may find it hard to stop. So, again, remember that you are aiming to get to -3 by your mealtime, when your body is telling you it wants something to eat.

You can try this next exercise when you are at that -3 point – once you've sorted out your eating routine (see Chapter 5) this should at a mealtime. It's about listening to the qualitative signals about what you have an appetite for. If this is something you haven't done for ages, it may take some learning, but that's fine. We'll take lunchtime at home on your own as an example.

From the favourite foods exercise earlier (see page 238), you have a few different lunch options. Bring one to mind and see it as clearly as you can. Imagine tasting it, and notice how much pleasurable feeling you get in your body. This feeling is what I call resonance. Now move on to visualizing option 2. Imagine tasting it and again notice how much pleasurable feeling you get. Then do the same with the other options.

You may find that one of the options has a stronger resonance right now, so go ahead and have that. Just the amount you've learned to judge by eye. So this lunch will be the size your body needs and the dish that you have an appetite for.

As an example, if you like the ingredients in the list on the left-hand side of the table below, you might love the combinations on the right. In this case, every lunchtime you'd bring each of the options on the right to mind, one at a time, and see which resonates most right now. And all the left-hand foods are simple things you can keep in stock at home.

Favourite foods	Lunch options
» Hummus and cheese » Favourite crackers » Loaf of favourite bread » Jar of peppers in olive oil » Jar of olives » Cherry tomatoes » Can of tuna	» Hummus and peppers on crackers » Cheese and tomato sandwich » Peppers, olives and tomatoes on toast » Tuna, pepper, olive and tomato salad

If it's mealtime but you can't tell which food seems most appealing right now, don't eat anything just yet. If you are trying to tune in to what your body wants and you can't tell, you probably aren't quite hungry enough yet. Wait for 5 or

10 minutes and then go back to asking yourself whether one type of food seems more appealing than the others. If you still can't tell then, make a guess and learn from how pleasurable it is whether your guess was a good one. If the food was disappointing and you still want to eat, that particular food didn't hit the spot and the skill needs more practice.

Using this skill will lead to you discover what you tend to like to eat at particular mealtimes and help you predict what you are likely to want, so you can buy the right foods when you're shopping. You may find that your tastes change from time to time, in which case you can easily adjust what you're buying to have available in your fridge and cupboards.

If you still can't tell then any food will satisfy the hunger (as opposed to the specific appetite), so just opt for any one of the possible lunches. Don't waste sweet or savoury snack foods in this case – if you can't tell, you might as well have something you love that is healthy.

If you really listen to your gut you will eat a balance of foods over time, even if not at each meal. Allow yourself the possibility of the one-food meal. This could be a (small) plate of a favourite vegetable, perhaps with your favourite sauce.

Do this exercise at any meal you have any influence over. If you're eating what someone else has cooked it's not likely to be an option, but that's okay. You don't have to eat just what you fancy every time, but the more you do, the more you will truly satisfy your appetite.

Dealing with sweet and savoury treats

If you're used to wanting to eat a lot of highly processed or manufactured foods, you may have been responding to the pleasure system in your brain rather than to your gut. Remember that those foods have been designed to be super-tasty and you may desire them irrespective of whether you are hungry. When you're not hungry, your gut isn't sending any what-to-eat signals, but your brain still remembers the 'bliss-point' foods and will urge you towards them if you even glimpse them.

When you're tempted to eat a sweet or savoury treat, the first step as ever is to tune in to where you are right now on the Appetite Pendulum™. If you aren't at -3, then it's not time to eat, so distract yourself away from food as you did in Chapter 7. If you are at -3, and you fancy eating the cake or chocolate bar, include that in the possible options for lunch.

In the early days of doing this you may find that your pleasure centre can't believe its luck, and that it shouts louder than your gut signals, and you opt for that as your lunch. But when you discover how fabulous things taste when they hit the spot, it won't always be cake that you fancy eating. Once the honeymoon of letting yourself eat cake is over, you'll find that your favourite 'real' lunch resonates more. When that happens, prepare yourself to be blown away. When you eat that fabulous real food for your lunch, when you're hungry, and you focus on eating it, you'll experience a quality of pleasure that knocks the spots off bought biscuits and cake. Truly. I mean, I have a very sweet tooth, but once I got into the swing of listening to what food was resonating with me, and ate that, I discovered that packets of bought biscuits and cake that I'd chosen in the past taste a bit weird. I think it's the flavour of the artificial sweeteners and preservatives coming through, and they no longer hold as much appeal at all. Well, I'm exaggerating a bit there – as the checkout staff at my local supermarket know, I'm not a total stranger to the sugary treats aisle.

Fabulous biscuits (M&S Extremely Chocolatey Milk Orange Chocolate Biscuits) and my favourite cake (Mary Berry's orange and sultana traybake) still do it for me, and I enjoy these more than ever. When I really fancy them, I have them and that is what I encourage you to do. But when you're being tempted by food that comes in a shiny wrapper, check with your gut whether that's what you really want.

'When you're not hungry, your gut isn't sending any what-to-eat signals, but your brain still remembers the "bliss-point" foods and will urge you towards them if you even glimpse them.'

Making sure what you eat tastes fabulous

As you retrain your appetite, you'll be eating less, so every mouthful needs to earn its place in your diet. To summarize what heightens pleasure when eating, here's my crib list:

1. Be definitely hungry
2. Have something you love
3. Have what resonates with your gut right now
4. Experiment with real food, freshly prepared, in season – and if you fancy a ready meal, have it and really enjoy it
5. Discover new foods and varieties and ways of cooking what you already love
6. Eat mindfully
7. Eat off heavy plates with heavy cutlery and drink from heavy glasses

And although we can't always control this, the situation we're in makes a big difference to the pleasurability of the meal. Talking and laughing can enhance the enjoyment of a meal, even if it distracts us a bit from the food. A tense unhappy meal can ruin even the finest cooking.

Eating snacks

The job of a snack is to tide you over between meals to stop you getting overly hungry. A snack should be small, so that it's digested before the next meal leaving you definitely hungry by that meal.

The snack you choose depends on how long it is until your next meal. If it's only 1–2 hours, then you want something that is going to be more quickly digested. Vegetables (raw, cooked, fresh or out of a jar or tin) are a good option and fruits such as a satsuma, pear or some grapes. If you've got two hours or more until your next meal, you'll need something more sustaining, like a small handful of nuts, a piece of cheese or a banana. Using trial and error you can discover what favourite snack keeps you going for how long, so you can take that with you if you know you're likely to need it.

Eating out

Eating out can be problematic when you are losing weight, but it doesn't need to be. The same principles of only starting to eat at -3 and stopping at +3 still apply and, if possible, keep to this when you dine out. In order to stop at +3, your task is to select what you really fancy from the menu, then eat with awareness of your fullness level and stop at +3. If there is food left on your plate, leave it. It may be that the amount you need to get you to +3 is a starter or a side dish or two. If you fancy a main course, then you may need to leave some of it. Special meals out don't mean weight gain when we eat just as much as our body needs rather than far too much

Problems stopping at +3 can arise when you want to get value for your money. For many people this means eating as much as possible of what they are served, but this search for value involves buying more than you need in the first place. Restaurants and other food outlets want you to spend as much as possible, so they offer you more food for relatively little more money. You spot a bargain and hey presto! You are eating far more than your body needs and if you eat out regularly, piling on pounds in the process. Instead, decide which food you want to buy, then eat only as much as you need to get to +3 and leave the rest. If you're worried about hurting the feelings of the waiting staff by leaving food on your plate, you can say that it was delicious but that you didn't need to eat all of it. When we eat what is put in front of us, we hand over control to other people to determine how much we eat. If their livelihood depends on serving us more, we will just go on getting fatter unless we tune in to our own bodies and listen to when to stop eating.

As you can see, Appetite Retraining saves you money when you are eating out just as when you eat at home, because you start to order less. You don't always need a side order. Indeed, if it is what you really fancy, you can just order a side order or two instead of a main course.

Once you arrive at your goal weight you will find that having an occasional meal out that is bigger than your normal meals will not lead you to put on weight – it's simply one meal and you will get back on track at the very next meal. Just as now, eating a bigger meal occasionally does not lead to weight gain any more than an occasional smaller meal leads you to lose weight.

'Single meals do not produce significant weight change; habitually large meals do.'

Plan ahead

It's a good idea to plan if you know you're going to be eating out. You want to arrive hungry, to get the most pleasure out of the food, so if the meal is later than your usual time, a really useful way to tide yourself over is with by having a vegetable-only meal. A smallish portion of your favourite vegetable can keep you going until the restaurant, by which time you'll have digested it and be heading towards -3 just in time.

Pressure from eating companions

So how can you deal with pressure from others over that celebratory meal that threatens to derail your newfound self-control? Or that business lunch that has all sorts of things riding on its success, leaving you feeling anxious and on edge?

There are different types of pressure. The genuine pressure from someone saying, 'I'll have one if you have one' or 'Are you going to have chips with that?' (in a tone of voice suggesting they want chips). Gradually you can learn to resist this sort of overt pressure by building your ability to say no. You can do this using Ronaldinho's technique (see page 93) by visualizing saying no in a friendly and firm way. This may not work immediately, particularly if you've caved in to this sort of pressure from this person before, but practice makes perfect and regular visualization can help.

If you're someone who tries to keep other people happy, you may feel imagined pressure from other people. 'S/he will feel better if I have dessert' or 'I need to order x to keep him/her happy.' Here what you need to develop is a slightly thicker skin when it comes to eating, so you focus on what your body wants, not what you think someone wants you to have. And remember you could be wrong anyway.

There's also the issue of polishing off what's on your plate to keep waiting staff and chefs happy. This is a tricky one. I once asked a client of mine who was an experienced chef whether chefs assume that if you left food on your plate you didn't like it. 'Of course, what else are we supposed to think?' was his reply. So there clearly is a risk that if you leave some of your dinner, the chef will be upset. Perhaps the best solution here is to ask for a takeaway box saying it was delicious and you want to have the rest later.

Sit-down restaurant meal

Menus aren't just thrown together; they are often carefully crafted and designed to draw you to ordering particular dishes. And in the buzz of a social event it's easy to chat at the expense of really looking at what's on the menu. In order to really enjoy this meal, and eat just the amount you want, breathe and relax. Tell yourself you have as much time as you need to look at the menu. Don't choose what appears low calorie or 'light' or choose on the basis of what other people are ordering.

Mentally, cross out any dish or any ingredient you don't like or can't eat. Look at what's left and see what resonates most by visualizing what the menu is telling you about each. Prepare to be surprised. What resonates most might be a starter or side or dessert. Take that as your first choice of what to have and then look at the rest of the menu to see what resonates most. If everyone else is having three courses, and you want to fit in, perhaps take into account what looks smaller, or plan to leave some.

Ask to see the dessert menu to help choose your whole meal. If the desserts that day don't really float your boat, plan to order coffee instead of dessert when the time comes.

When the food arrives, focus on enjoying your food through all five senses. Notice how the dish looks and smells, the tastes and textures. All that sensory information is adding to your pleasure.

As you eat, if you can, notice your Appetite Pendulum™ number. Eat the best bits of each course and leave the less tasty bits, risking the wrath of the kitchen. Or take your own takeaway box with you and take what you don't eat away and throw it away.

When it comes to dessert, if you're already at +3 or more then it's a good idea to order a hot drink and a dessert with a takeaway box (if dessert is included in the price). If you do still fancy dessert, eat it mindfully perhaps just having a few bites and take the rest with you. Note that you might enjoy this dessert more if you eat it tomorrow.

Shun the bread basket

Unless bread is going to be one of the best bits of your meal, decline it. It will dull your taste buds and can easily get you to +3 before anything you've ordered reaches your table. It doesn't matter whether it's free. I carry food bags with me for situations like this, and sneak the bread home with me for another day.

The all-you-can-eat buffet

Faced with an enormous fabulous-looking spread, and loving a bargain, we are prey to piling our plates and going back for more when an all-you-can-eat buffet is on offer. But eating as much as you can is only a bargain if you want to gain weight, in which case the all-you-can-eat buffet is your friend. The two-pronged problem is the amount and the variety of what's in front of you at the buffet spread, leaving you overwhelmed by choice. Here is how to handle the buffet using Appetite Retraining:

» Arrive hungry (or on the way to being -3 if you think there will be a long pre-amble to the meal).

» Plan the size and timing of your previous meal to allow this, perhaps with a veg-only meal at your usual dinner time.

» Choose to sit as far away from the buffet as you can and

with your back to it, so that you're less tempted to go back for more.

» Limit the number of different foods you choose to three, and opt for your real favourites. Taste-specific satiety (see page 52) means that although your taste buds lose their sensitivity as you eat bite by bite, each new dish refreshes your appetite. This means that it's easier to stop eating if you limit how many different things you have on your plate – if you choose five dishes you'll taste them all whether you're still hungry or not.

» Remember to maximize enjoyment, not intake – quality and taste over quantity every time.

» Give the bread basket a wide berth unless it's in your top three.

» Eat mindfully using all five senses (see page 96).

» Leave what you don't like.

» Take a takeaway box with you (this way you can feel you've got better value for money).

» Remember what I said about the issue of waste (see page 105). Food is no less wasted when it goes through our body then into the toilet than when it goes straight into the recycling bin. When you get to +3 (or +4 for a special meal if you prefer) leave what's left or take it with you. That way it won't be stored as fat.

'If you're trying to eat in tune with your body, the all-you-can-eat buffet is the demonic twin of the free bar!'

Fast food joints

If your weakness is for a burger and chips, you can still retrain your appetite without giving this up. When you visit your favourite fast food outlet, find a smaller version of what you usually have. The best options here are often the kids' meals. That way you can get a smaller drink, smaller burger (or whatever), smaller fries and discover how much of the kids' meal you need to eat to get to +3. You may be surprised to discover (as I did to my astonishment) that even a kids' meal is more than enough. Once you've worked it out you can order exactly the right amount, saving money, losing weight and reducing food waste all at one fell swoop.

Then the usual principles apply as for any meal out: arrive hungry, choose your favourite thing(s), eat mindfully, stop at +3 and throw the rest away.

Take-aways

I'm almost embarrassed to tell you what I've discovered about takeaways. Until I retrained my own appetite, I always had the same Indian takeaway: chicken korma, saag bhajee and plain naan. I didn't bother with rice because I preferred naan. Once I started on my own appetite retraining quest, I started really noticing how much of this usual takeaway got me to +3.

The simple answer is 'not very much'. In fact, as with all my other meals, it was astonishingly little. So I started focusing more on which of the takeaway dishes I liked best and discovered that, hands down, it was the saag bhajee. To cut a medium length story short, what transpired was that my ideal (seriously) Indian takeaway is now a side portion of saag bhajee. Nothing else. If I feel like it, I order some korma sauce (no chicken – just the sauce) to go with it, but usually I just want the saag. It tastes sublime, it gets me to my +3 and I feel great afterwards. Gone is that unpleasant slightly drugged feeling that came 20 minutes after my old-style takeaway, and I'm then just hungry enough for my 9.30pm snack.

My old takeaway cost me £12.60 a time; the new one is £3.50. Add a couple of quid on the korma sauce days. Unfortunately my favourite Indian has closed down recently. I hope it wasn't due to loss of revenue from me.

You can use the same approach to retraining your takeaway habit. Start with what you order now, and step by step discover your favourite dishes so that you can start buying less. If you usually share your takeaway with someone else, you could share a single portion of anything you usually buy two of, and so on.

What to do with the money you save!
If you work out how much less you've forked out for each meal out or takeaway, you can start a savings jar with the money you save each time. You may be surprised at how much this is. You can decide how to spend it – on a pampering treat or buying yourself something for your home that you've hankered after. Or you can treat yourself to a

fabulous meal out. No reason why you can't spend that extra money on lovely food.

Whatever you choose to spend it on, notice that every month, you'll continue saving the same amount, and you can keep going with spending that on treats, or just enjoy the fact that there's now less of your monthly budget spent on food you didn't need and wouldn't really have enjoyed!

As you've been retraining your appetite one step at a time throughout this book, the next question is how to maintain your new weight once you arrive at your goal. In the next chapter I'll show you how the work you've already done on making stepwise changes to your eating habits was the hard bit and that sticking to your new weight is easy. There will of course be challenges, such as holidays, and we'll look at how to deal with those.

CHAPTER 10

—

Maintain Your New Weight

The weight you settle at might not be what you aimed for in the first place. Many people I've worked with have started with a particular goal on the scales but over weeks and months of making changes, their ambitions change. Often they expand their view of what 'happy with myself' will look like, so it's much more about being flexibly in control around eating instead of feeling out of control. Or they realize that feeling comfortable in their own skin is what matters to them and that means a shift in self-acceptance and self-love rather than a shift on the dial.

Whatever weight you settle at, the absolute essential is that eating is easy and joyful. Remember that what we weigh is in large part because of our eating habits. You're going to be eating like this for the rest of your life. Your new habits need to be ones that fill you with confidence and really delicious food, so if to get to a lower point on the scales than you've got to means forgoing a lot in terms of eating-pleasure, think about staying at this level at least for the time being. In the months ahead, if you feel like making another change and you have the energy and mental bandwidth to do it, you can make that next change.

> '**Whaever weight you settle at, the absolute essential is that eating is easy and joyful. Your new habits need to be ones that fill you with confidence and really delicious food.**'

Maintaining your new habits (is easy)

The more you do the new thing, the more automatic it becomes – that's what habits are – and soon it will be easier to do the new thing than the old. The hard work you put in to making the changes will now be paying off. Your new eating habits are the eating habits that sustain the weight you've arrived at and when you stick to these new habits, your weight will stay stable.

You're likely to find that at times, you're inclined to do the old thing (like have seconds though you're already +3), but this isn't a problem as long as you decide whether this is a special occasion on which you choose to do this. Or decide that you're better off sticking to the new pattern.

Remember to keep your focus on maximizing the pleasure you're getting from food, by eating just enough at this meal so you get definitely hungry by the next, as well as choosing your favourite foods, and experimenting with new tastes and combinations. Choose the best food you can afford and if you need to, go on a cookery course. I went on a one-evening how-to-cook-curry course at the Square Food Foundation in Bristol because I didn't know my way around Indian spices or how to use them. One single evening, and I now know enough to make saag aloo (a new favourite) and chicken korma myself. OK, so I haven't gone far from the korma and spinach routine, but cooking it from scratch is a pleasure in itself.

Exercise and movement

There's a growing consensus that exercise in itself is an ineffective way to lose weight. It's changing how you eat that makes the difference to what you weigh. But when you start losing weight, you're likely to find that you want to move around more, and there are good reasons to do so. One is that the health benefits of exercise are phenomenal. Another is that people who exercise regularly tend to maintain weight loss.

So make it easier on yourself to stay on track by finding the ways your body most likes to move around. Choose something that is fun like dancing or Zumba, or that gives you an endorphin rush like running or cycling, or that you can do with friends like badminton, walking or swimming. If you enjoy it, you're more likely to do it again. And it's the regularity that helps.

You can look in to what combination of duration and intensity suits you. High Intensity Interval Training that you do at home might suit you if you have a lot of commitments at home or have a very busy job with virtually no time to call your own. A sociable visit to the gym with coffee afterwards might be more up your street if you have more time.

Going off track and how to get back on track

While you are in the process of changing the eating habits of a lifetime, you may find that you veer off course occasionally and it may take quite a lot of energy and focus to get back on track. The main thing is to realize that you're going to have to hold tight and steer your way back to your new focus, and that this will take extra effort, but only briefly. Remind yourself that all that's happened is that you've gone off track and that you can get back on course again by reminding yourself of your Best Benefit (see page 74) and putting your mental energy into resuming your new habits.

Because of the effort involved, you'll probably find it easier to keep on track in the first place, by noticing any temptation to revert to an old habit and focusing hard on your Best Benefit and the fact that you can choose at the moment of temptation to go ahead or to go backwards.

Each time you keep on track despite temptation to go backwards, and each time you bring yourself back on course after veering off, notice what it tells you about yourself that you managed to do this. It might show you that you can be strong, determined, resilient or resourceful. Whatever it is, it's part of your new identity and self-image, and something to be proud of.

High days, holidays and festivities

Days of celebration often mean communal meals, and large ones at that. They don't come round all that often, so when you've arrived at a comfortable weight and your eating habits are easy to stick to, you can splash out for a day without gaining weight. You may gain a couple of pounds on the scales that day, but these will be quickly lost again when you resume your new eating patterns.

Then there are the festive seasons, such as Christmas and New Year, where there may be one huge meal after another towering buffet. This is more of a challenge than the single day, so requires a bit more planning. One way to deal with it is to stick to your new eating habits at all of these parties, just choosing exactly what you want from the menu or buffet and then heading for the dance floor to move away from food. Or you could decide which special events you'd like to push the boat out for, and balance the day overall by having lighter meals or snacks the rest of the time.

Holidays are much like festive seasons writ large, when it may be tempting to indulge at every meal either because you're trying to get your money's worth, or simply because you're on holiday. Here we go back to the points about the all-you-can-eat buffet (which may be what you are actually faced with at every meal if you're on a cruise or in a hotel with an inclusive package). Think quality instead, and limit how many different tastes you have at each meal. And perhaps, notice what it feels like to walk away from the buffet with a smallish plate of fabulous food while you notice other people piling their plates high. It may help you realize that you can control your eating, even at a 'free' buffet, and how many of us ever regret not eating something half an hour later?

By having just what your body needs, you can arrive home the same weight as when you left, having had a relaxing, enjoyable and confidence-building holiday.

> **'If you're trying to lose weight, quantity over quality is *not* value for money. It means you buying exactly what you don't want.'**

Adjusting to your new body and sense of self

When we start to look different, mental energy is required to adjust to our new appearance. Looking in the mirror will be a mini-surprise each time you do it and other people may look at you differently. This may all come as a welcome relief, but it may also take some getting used to.

I suggest that you look in the mirror regularly as you lose weight and get used to your appearance changing. You might want to buy the occasional item of clothing, though it would make sense to wait until you've got where you want to get to before overhauling your wardrobe. When you are ready to take that step, get your favourite clothes taken in both to save money and to avoid having to part with lovely garments.

When you're shopping for clothes take various sizes into the changing room, and see which fits you best. You won't necessarily know. Your top and bottom halves may have changed size to different extents, and it's easy to dismiss the idea that you could actually be a few clothes sizes smaller now.

Talk to yourself regularly about your progress, and about what you're learning about yourself. You need to update your emotional/psychological view of yourself, not just how you look in the mirror. Say to yourself, 'I can gauge what my body needs' or 'I can achieve my goal even though I doubted it' or whatever is right for you. And keep saying these things to remind yourself of what you're discovering about yourself.

Finally, you'll need to tolerate the weirdness of achieving your goal, particularly if you've tried and failed to get here many times before. I feel quite emotional writing this, because I've seen many people who have gained so much more from retraining their appetite than just what they lost on the scales. They've done it themselves. Not me. I haven't checked their trolley at the supermarket, or hidden their chocolate. Many of them have used Appetite Retraining as a stepping stone to developing their own way of eating and being around food. And they've all discovered that by retraining your appetite you can get more joy from food than you ever did before.

—

Resources

References

Callahan, R.J. (2001), *Tapping the Healer Within*. McGraw Hill

Enders, G (2014), *Gut: The Inside Story of our body's most under-rated organ*. Scribe

Fairburn, C.G. (2013), *Overcoming Binge Eating*. 2nd edition. Guilford Press

Fletcher, H (1906), *The New Glutton or Epicure*. B.F. Stevens & Brown

Guilano, Mireille (2005), *French Women Don't Get Fat: The Secret of Eating for Pleasure*. Vintage Books

Hopkinson, S and Bareham, L (1997), *The Prawn Cocktail Years*. Macmillan

Kessler, D.A. (2009), *The End of Overeating*. Penguin

Mischel, W (2014), *The Marshmallow Test*. Corgi

Mosley, M (2015), *The 8-Week Blood Sugar Diet*. Short Books

Pearson, L and Pearson, L (1973), *The Psychologist's Eat-Anything Diet*. Gestalt Journal Press

Reid, S (2008) *The Amazing Adventures of Diet Girl*. Corgi

Shapiro, F. (2012) *Getting Past Your Past*. Rodale

Shapiro, R. (2005) The Two-Hand Interweave in Shapiro, R. *EMDR Solutions: Pathways to Healing*. Norton

Spector, T (2015) *The Diet Myth*. Weidenfeld and Nicolson

Spence, C (2018) *Gastrophysics: The New Science of Eating*. Penguin

Further reading

If you are suffering from post-traumatic stress, Claudia Herbert's book *Overcoming Traumatic Stress* (2nd edition) is a compassionately written, comprehensive guide to recovering from psychological trauma which explains why you're experiencing the symptoms you have, and how to deal with each of them.

For help dealing with very intense emotions try the book *The Mindfulness Solution for Intense Emotions: Take Control of Borderline Personality Disorder with DBT* by Cedar Koons.

For a self-help book on overcoming eating disorders, Carolyn Costin and Gwen Grabb's book 8 *Keys to Recovery from an Eating Disorder* is extremely helpful. The authors combine professional expertise with personal experience of overcoming an eating disorder.

Psychological therapy and counselling

If you're looking for professional help with issues that are linked with eating more than you want to, such as low self-esteem or finding it hard to regulate your emotions without food, there are many approaches that can help. Each of us is different, and what helps one person may not help another. If you're looking for therapy, the individual therapist may or may not be someone you feel you can work with, and you should trust your judgement on this. Your first port of call may be your GP who can tell you about local services in the NHS, voluntary sector and private sector. Not all therapies are available on the NHS.

There are many forms of therapeutic help. Perhaps the best known is cognitive-behavioural therapy (CBT) which looks at how your patterns of thinking and behaving may be maintaining your difficulties, and helps you change them. There are new approaches related to CBT such as Acceptance and Commitment Therapy and Compassion-Focused Therapy.

Insight-oriented psychotherapies focus on helping you identify patterns of relating to yourself and others which were established in your early life, so that by understanding these patterns, you can change them. These include approaches that developed from psycho-analysis and include Psychodynamic Psychotherapy.

Approaches to reducing distress which work physically on the body work best for some people, as they focus more on the physical manifestations of distress and require less talking about the problem. Eye Movement Desensitization and Reprocessing (EMDR) uses a clear and carefully-followed protocol for working through unresolved traumatic memories through the use of bilateral stimulation. This can be helpful if you're suffering from a problem which has its roots in a traumatic event (or multiple traumatic events).

Other body-based approaches include Sensorimotor Psychotherapy and Somatic Experiencing. Energy Therapy approaches such as the Emotional Freedom Technique (EFT) and Thought Field Therapy (TFT) are gentle and for some, powerful ways to reduce distressing symptoms and emotions.

Diagnostic Criteria for Binge Eating Disorder

From the *Diagnostic and Statistical Manual of Mental Disorders* – Fifth Edition (DSM-5)

A. Recurrent episodes of binge eating. An episode of binge eating is characterised by both of the following:
1. Eating, in a discrete period of time (e.g. within any 2-hour period), an amount of food that is definitely larger than what most people would eat in a similar period of time under similar circumstances.
2. A sense of lack of control over eating during the episode (e.g. a feeling that one cannot stop eating or control how much one is eating).

B. The binge-eating episodes are associated with three (or more) of the following:
1. Eating much more rapidly than normal
2. Eating until feeling uncomfortably full
3. Eating large amounts of food when not feeling physically hungry
4. Eating alone because of feeling embarrassed by how much one is eating
5. Feeling disgusted with oneself, depressed or very guilty afterward

C. Marked distress regarding binge eating is present.

D. The binge eating occurs, on average, at least once a week for three months.

E. The binge eating is not associated with the recurrent use of inappropriate compensatory behaviour as in bulimia nervosa and does not occur exclusively during the course of bulimia nervosa or anorexia nervosa.

Level of severity:
Mild: 1–3 binge eating episodes per week
Moderate: 4–7 binge eating episodes per week
Severe: 8–13 binge eating episodes per week
Extreme: 14 or more binge-eating episodes per week

Useful organizations

British Association for Behavioural and Cognitive Psychotherapies (lists therapists qualified to provide CBT) **www.babcp.com**

British Psychological Society (lists qualified Clinical Psychologists and Counselling Psychologists) **www.bps.org.uk**

British Psychoanalytic Council (lists psychodynamic and psychoanalytic psychotherapists) **www.bpc.org.uk**

Emotional Freedom Technique (lists practitioners trained in EFT, a form of Energy Therapy) **www.emofree.com**

Eye Movement Desensitization and Reprocessing Association of UK and Ireland (lists professionals qualified to provide EMDR) **www.emdrassociation.org.uk**

UK Council for Psychotherapy (lists psychotherapists and psychotherapeutic counsellors) **www.psychotherapy.org.uk**

Other useful websites and resources

BEAT Eating Disorders is a charity that provides advice about eating disorders **www.beateatingdisorders.org.uk**

Mark Grant's website **www.overcomingpain.com** has a link to the App 'Anxiety Release with Bilateral Stimulation' and an App to help you sleep called 'Sleep Restore'

Thought Field Therapy (Dr Callahan's website which includes some free materials) **www.tfttapping.com**

Acknowledgements

By the time I started to work on Appetite Retraining in 2011 I'd learned a great deal from colleagues and supervisors over the years who had shaped and spurred on my professional development. To start with I was extremely lucky to be supervised in Oxford by Professor Gordon Claridge, Professor David Clarke and the late Dr William Parry-Jones, all of whom taught me a huge amount about clinically relevant research and made my D.Phil. research interesting, challenging and fun.

I then had an enormously positive experience of being trained in Clinical Psychology on the South-East Thames In-Service Training Scheme led by Professor Tony Lavender. I was extremely fortunate to land my first post-qualification job in the Clinical Psychology Department of Oxleas NHS Trust, supervised by David Walker. I learned a huge amount about putting psychology into practice to help people from David, Tony, my colleagues and supervisors.

Developing Appetite Retraining meant starting with a goal, but having absolutely no idea how to achieve it. The person who has helped me most, at each and every step of this process is my husband Gerard McCarthy. He has encouraged and supported me throughout with discussions, suggestions, insights and when all else failed, humour. Without him I'd have given up long ago. Our children Betsy and Edward egged me on and made fun of me in equal measure, as my own meals got smaller and I became increasingly fussy about eating only my very favourite foods!

I've had extremely helpful input along the way from my friends Hazel Bedford, Kate Berkeley, Irene Inskip, Dr Elisabeth Marx and Dr Jane Midforth.

The staff at Litfield House Medical Centre in Bristol and Cyncoed Consulting Rooms in Cardiff have been extremely supportive and helpful both practically and in friendship. I am particularly grateful to Trisha Tanner who helped me develop my practice in Bristol.

Sonja Jefferson and Sharon Tanton showed me how to present what I was doing in writing and online. With additional help from Pam Lloyd, Sue Richardson and Kelly Mundt-Czerkawska I was then able to produce the outline of this book. Iain Claridge designed my website, Eliza Bott designed the logo and the Appetite Pendulum™, and Claire Rees is helping me with PR.

I am delighted that it was Pavilion Books who took me on. I'm eternally grateful to David Graham, Katie Cowan and Steph Milner who gave me this opportunity to get my work into print. Steph oversaw the whole process and guided me skilfully through it, and Dawn Bates worked on the manuscript with me, and greatly improved the structure and flow of the book.

I owe a lot to all the clients who have worked with me over the years as they have taught me a great deal about how to change, and it is through working with them that I've learned about overcoming hurdles to change.

Finally I'd like to say thank you to all the Bristol GPs who were enthusiastic and encouraging about Appetite Retraining, and who kept asking when I'd write a book. Here it finally is!

INDEX

—